STOP OVERTHINKING

A PRACTICAL GUIDE TO FINDING PEACE OF MIND AND LETTING GO

MIA PARKER

TABLE OF CONTENTS

INTRODUCTION & MY STORY

To think too much is a disease. –Fyodor Dostoevsky

Are you completely exhausted at the end of the day? Are your eyelids impossible to keep open? Do you feel like you could sleep for days, but when your head hits the pillow, your brain kicks into overdrive? Do you watch your day in rewind like reruns of an old TV show and replay every scene word for word? *Did I really say that to my boss? I can't believe I wore white shoes today—it's still December! Did I lock the front door?* Or maybe you go back a few years, like to that day in high school when you walked past the football players with toilet paper stuck to your shoe.

My face still flushes over that last one! Like you, I used to overthink—*everything.* Hi! I'm Mia, recovering overthinker.

On my way to becoming a finance executive and CFO for a major U.S. corporation, I developed new strengths at every turn. Those skills got me to the corner office, but by the time I got there, I was in turmoil. I suffered constant anxiety from overthinking every meeting and, really, every sentence I heard from my coworkers.

When I first started my career, I was the only woman in the finance department. I felt like I had to prove myself every day and work twice as hard as my male counterparts in order to be taken seriously. One day, during a meeting, my coworker John interrupted me and took credit for my idea. I was furious and wanted to call him out, but I knew that as a woman, I had to tread carefully. *I'm going to march right in there and give him a piece of my mind. No, I'll just sound like the whiny woman they think doesn't belong in the corporate world. I'll be passive-aggressive and let John know that I know what he did, but the boss doesn't know what he did or know that I know what he did, and I'm going to hold that over John's head. No! That's not passive-aggressive; it's blackmail. Um… I'll just go directly to the boss and claim my work. Maybe. What if he thinks I'm tattling? That will just confirm I'm a whiny woman who doesn't belong in the corporate world.* After overthinking the whole scenario, playing it out in my head and worrying about possible outcomes, thinking I knew beforehand what both John and my boss thought, wasting a lot of precious time and energy, and driving myself nearly over the edge, I took a deep breath and calmly pointed out to John that it was actually my idea. I didn't make a big scene, but I made sure that I was heard. Later on, I brought up the incident with my boss and explained how it made me feel. He listened and acknowledged that there was a problem. We worked together to establish more equitable communication norms for our team, and it made a big difference.

My excessive thoughts did not lead me to any solution. They kept me paralyzed in fear of what-ifs and anxious over every possibility I entertained. I got mad at myself for squandering so much time I could have used to be productive that afternoon, and I ruminated over it even more when I got home from work that evening. *I should have spoken up sooner. I should have said {this} instead of {that}.*

I should have been assertive during the meeting and claimed my work. Oh! I just thought of the best insult for John, that purloining, plagiarizing egotist! The return to these thoughts took my attention away from my husband, who hadn't had the best day himself. He probably had some choice words about me and my neglect of our relationship in his internal dialogue.

Although I kept a cool exterior, it was all a facade. My inner world and my personal life were quietly crumbling.

When my marriage broke down, and after my emotional state revealed itself, I left my career to focus on myself, and through studies in psychology and mindfulness, I discovered a pathway to fixing myself. And guess what? I finally found happiness.

On my journey, I found that many women suffer from the same anxieties I did. Now, my goal is to put my experiences to work and help you find the relief and peace—and sanity—that I now reside in. I hope you will let this book be your guide. In it, we will consider the following:

- what overthinking is and why it's a common problem
- the negative effects of overthinking on mental and physical health
- effective strategies to overcome this challenge and to *Stop Overthinking*

WHAT IS OVERTHINKING?

Overthinking is pretty easy to define. It means to, well, overthink. It means that even though you've moved on from one subject to another, you keep rehashing the first one. Not only that, but you'll remember an old conversation you had with a friend and *really* wish you had said this other thing. Or maybe you finally remember the punchline to the joke you wanted to tell your dad. Your mind mulls it over: *Boy, he would have liked that one! I'll have to call him later. Hope I still remember the joke then. Oh! It will be even funnier if I tell it this way…* You might even start analyzing your grocery list, planning your next vacation, and solving all the world's problems. A lot of these things can't be changed because they're in the past or because you simply have no power to do anything (like solve the world's problems). Some, however, may be doable, but the problem is that you're not letting them out of your head.

Here's the kicker: You bring the stress of overthinking upon yourself. Instead of taking action on what you're contemplating, you just keep going over it and over it. When you get stuck in the loop, you get nothing accomplished. It can affect your success at your job because you're not focusing on the tasks in front of you. It can destroy relationships—I know from experience—because you're not focused on your partner but on the trivial things in your mind. It can really make you anxious because you're not accomplishing the things you're thinking about despite thinking about them so thoroughly, and this can result in depression because you feel like a failure for not getting these things resolved (and for not solving the world's problems).

There Is Hope!

I know you long for peace of mind. You want to get off the roller coaster of emotion and frustration. You want to be productive again. In the chapters ahead, we'll dive into techniques that can help you do just that.

Some helpful solutions we'll discuss are

- realizing when you're stuck in a loop
- shifting your focus
- applying mindfulness practices
- learning to emotionally detach from your own thoughts

I'm grateful that you've picked up this book, and I'm proud of you for taking this step toward regaining control of your thoughts. My hope for you is that by the end of the book, you will have rediscovered *you* and that you will understand how to help yourself and others who find themselves caught in a similar mind trap. Let's get started, shall we?

CHAPTER 1:
UNDERSTANDING OVERTHINKING

STOP OVERTHINKING

MIA PARKER

Man is not worried by real problems so much as by his imagined anxieties about real problems. –Epictetus

Whether you know it or not, if you're an overthinker, your happiness is being compromised daily. As mentioned in the Introduction, it's a very unhealthy habit, both mentally and physically. Although overthinking is not recognized as a mental health condition, it is symptomatic of anxiety and depression. Actually, it's not really known which causes which; it's a bit of a chicken-or-egg quandary. What experts do know, however, is that it can be eased, and your happiness can once again bubble over.

As we learn more about this overthinking conundrum, keep these two points in mind (Sperber, n.d.):

- **You overthink to protect yourself.** This may add to the conundrum aspect, but think about it—for right now, of course, and then let it go and move on to the next point. I jest, but seriously, the thoughts you ruminate over usually begin as something that's important to you. Maybe you need to resolve a financial issue, or perhaps you have to figure out what keeps tripping the fuse to your electrical outlet. These issues are important and valid. You want to avoid money problems, and you don't want your appliances to short out. These are real concerns that require real solutions. Your mind is trying to work them out and bring you relief, but it just can't seem to stop when it lands on a good plan.

- **You do not intentionally overthink.** Most thoughts happen automatically. You don't get in bed and tell yourself to ruminate. *Okay, it's 10 p.m. now, and my alarm is set for 6 a.m. That gives me a full eight hours to drive myself crazy! I have an important meeting with a client tomorrow, so I will think about the presentation and the various ways it can and will fail and how I'll lose my job over it and…*

Despite its good intentions and innate routines, your mind may still get stuck in a rut.

YOU'VE GOT TO KNOW WHAT IT IS BEFORE YOU CAN DEFEAT IT

To get a better understanding of what we're dealing with, let's take a look at the official definition of "overthinking" according to the Merriam-Webster dictionary: "to think too much about (something) : to put too much time into thinking about or analyzing (something) in a way that is more harmful than helpful" (n.d.-d).

Not sure if you're an overthinker or just a heavy thinker? Take a look at this checklist. Mark all that apply:

You have a lot of negative thoughts.

You feel like you can't turn your brain off.

You are mentally exhausted.

You are often physically exhausted.

You are unable to relax.

You struggle to make decisions.

You second-guess every decision you do make.

Once you make and carry out a decision, you expect it to fail.

You view every potential outcome as the worst possible scenario.

You are relentlessly anxious.

You are often depressed.

Once you start thinking about something, you are unable to stop.

Once you start thinking about something, you can think of nothing else.

What you think about often takes a tangent and ends up back where you started.

You replay past events and conversations in your mind.

You sleep fewer than six hours per night (and even that's a stretch).

You struggle to focus on important tasks at hand.

You find it difficult to pay attention during conversations because your thoughts are consuming you.

You obsess over day-to-day interactions with friends, coworkers, or family members.

You read into words and actions things that aren't really there.

You fixate on what you cannot control.

If you checked the majority—or all—of the boxes, welcome to the club you didn't really want to join.

Sarah Sperber of the Berkley Well-Being Institute refines Merriam-Webster's definition and describes overthinking as "the process of repetitive, unproductive thought" (n.d.). She goes on to explain that thoughts cannot be focused on multiple things at once. That's why the subject that first consumes you eventually morphs into another area of concern. She says researchers refer to the times when you overthink a past or present occurrence as "rumination," and they call it "worry" when your focus is on something that may (or may not) happen in the future. Any time you dwell on an issue, like repeatedly replaying a conversation or event that ended badly in your mind, focusing solely on your shortcomings or failures, and reliving your mistakes in your mind, you are putting your mental health at risk. With mental health decline comes more rumination, and your ability to end the cycle weakens.

I agree with Merriam-Webster's description. Overthinking is definitely not helpful! It's quite the oxymoron, isn't it? You'd think that thinking would be helpful, but when you can't stop thinking about what you're thinking about, no decisions get made, no actions get taken, and no peace gets to your mind.

When I was an overthinker, I stayed awake hours one night excessively analyzing my family tree. We had traced the surname back to the 1550s. The youngest members of our family right now are the 14th generation from that person. All night long, I kept thinking about each of the men in the line of progression. Before my head hit the pillow, I could list each one—all 13 of them in order! But as I lay there, I rethought the list. And then I rethought it again because I was missing someone. *Aha! Got it!* I rethought the list again, but I was missing someone else that time. *Aha! Got it!* And on it went. It was like trying to name the seven dwarfs: You always forget one. I finally got to the point of naming all 13 men in order again, and I thought I would be able to sleep. Nope! Then, I was suddenly starving. And I wondered what #10 in that family tree would have eaten if he got hungry at 3 a.m. That rolled into what #9 would eat, and #8, and then I wondered why I started with guy #10, so I went back to the end and pondered guy #13, then #12, then #11, then skipped #10, #9, and #8, because I'd already thought about them, but then I didn't feel right about messing up the list so I reviewed them anyway.

Needless to say, I was useless at work the next day. I was not only physically exhausted from lack of sleep, but my brain was worn out from running overtime on nothing important. I missed deadlines that day and had to cancel meetings because I could not think. That is, I could not actively think about what was important—the things that actually mattered to my career and my life in general. Ironic, huh?

Overthinking Is Not Problem-Solving

Some people dismiss overthinking as problem-solving. They claim they aren't wasting precious intellectual time because they are trying to find a solution to a particular issue. If that were as far as it went, that would be okay, but the real problem that needs to be solved is how to stop thinking once you've found the answer you were looking for. Overthinking goes beyond problem-solving when the analytical process takes over and moves on to tangents. This is demonstrated by my overnight family tree rumination. I should have been able to sleep once I solved the problem of listing all the men in order, but a hunger pang sent me on a side trip to revisit the list another way.

Problem-solving is actually a very valuable skill. We all encounter problems every day. Let's consider this very minor problem as an example: It's Saturday morning, and your friends are coming over for brunch, but you forgot to stop at the grocery store yesterday, and you have nothing to serve them. What do you do?

A person with a healthy mindset would either make a quick run for supplies, be creative with what's on hand, order food to be delivered, or send a mass text to their friends and ask them each to bring something. That's a successful problem-solver:

- They realized there was a problem.
- They brainstormed possible solutions.

- They stopped thinking about it when they came to one that would work.
- They put the solution to task, and they moved on from the problem.

What would you—an overthinker—do? You would do steps one, two, and maybe three (briefly) above, but when you arrived at four, you would not move on. You would ruminate first over the dilemma, then over each option. In the end, you may not even arrive at a decision and could be completely unprepared when your friends start to arrive. At that point, you'd be embarrassed and devastated. Though you may keep a calm appearance, your anxiety would boil over, and depression would later follow. Your friends would probably tease and laugh it off and decide *for you* that you should all go out to eat and make you foot the bill. You're so relieved you could cry, and later that day after your friends have all gone home, you will—while you rehash the whole situation and consider what you should have done differently and hope your friends will continue to be your friends.

When you overthink, you don't solve anything; rather, you tend to create more problems. As registered psychotherapist Natacha Duke aptly describes, "You get caught up in the thinking loop and you end up where you started. In some cases, you may even end up with more worry and anxiety" (*Overthinking Disorder*, 2022). Problem-solving moves you forward, but overthinking paralyzes you.

Types of Overthinking

I think we can agree that problem-solving is not a type of overthinking. It is more like a goal to strive for as you learn to overcome this challenge that plagues you. That's one thing this book aims to help you achieve: to recognize when you've reached the solution, halt the thought process, and take action on that plan.

You might think overthinking is overthinking and that your brain runs on overtime no matter how you look at it, but there are actually different types. *Verywell Mind* lists three common ones (Morin, 2023b):

- **Overgeneralizing:** In this case, you base all future events on the outcome of one particular past occasion. Let's say the back of your gown was tucked into your underwear when you walked down the aisle as a bridesmaid at your friend's wedding. (Yes, I borrowed that from *Friends!*) So you decide to stop wearing dresses of all sorts because any dress or skirt or skirt-like pants or clothing item could potentially get stuck like that—and most definitely *will* get stuck *every* single time you ever attempt to wear something like that in the future—and expose your backside to the entire world.

- **All-or-nothing:** There's no happy medium in this type of thinking. Everything is black or white, good or bad, positive or negative, will work out for good or will work out for evil. You analyze, reanalyze, and overanalyze every potential outcome of a situation as either a complete success or a complete failure. Either way, it stresses you out because even a success could have its flaws that you would surely look back on and ruminate about.

- **Catastrophizing:** This type of thinking sets you up for failure before you even have a chance to give an opportunity a try. I had a friend like this. He found himself out of work unexpectedly, so he hit the job boards to see what was available for someone with his skill level, education, and career experience. Every time he found something interesting, though, he had himself fired before he even applied! Catastrophizing means worrying you will fail at something, then thinking through the event and seeing yourself fail at each step along the way, only to find yourself in the worst-case scenario—the unrealistic worst-case scenario.

Each type is a result of what experts call cognitive distortions. These usually negative thoughts are driven by irrational ways of thinking. They leave you unmotivated, tank your self-esteem, and can even lead to mental health issues as well as substance misuse and addictions.

You may tend toward one or all of the above.

WHAT CAUSES OVERTHINKING?

Why are some people able to determine a thought process is over while others get stuck in the loop? Some people may just be more naturally inclined to overthink. It's unclear if the tendency is genetic or learned. You may battle the habit because a parent also contended with it and passed the inclination on to you in your DNA, or you could have seen it modeled to you growing up, and the behavior led you to mimic your parent's incessant ponderings. Whatever the cause, you are not alone in the struggle. The latest research tallies show 73% of people 25–35 years old and 52% of people aged 45–55 are chronic cogitators (Santilli, 2023).

As mentioned earlier, overthinking is often associated with anxiety and depression. Some experts blame PTSD, but you don't have to have had a traumatic experience or experienced a crisis to develop this habit. Even the mere suggestion of something can send you over the edge.

When I was an overthinker, it wasn't just trivial things that caught me in a loop. If I felt a strange health symptom and went to Dr. Google—you guessed it! I was dying. One time, I noticed what I interpreted to be a heart palpitation. I thought, *Oh no! Is that normal? Does that happen to everybody, like healthy people? Is my heart okay? Am I going to have to go to the doctor over this? Should I go to the doctor? Would it be stupid to just let it go? Can I just let it go? It's my heart!* I happen to have a finger monitor in the bathroom closet, so I put that on, and lo and behold, the heart rate was uneven! It was jumping up and down and *Was that a flatline?* and going jagged. I went back to wondering *Is this okay? Am I having a heart attack? Will I have a heart attack if I don't go to the doctor right now? I should go to the doctor. It'll be fine. Wait. Let me check these other things. Nope! I don't have the other symptoms Dr. Google describes. I don't want to go to the doctor. The thought of that makes me extra anxious! And what if they find something? Even though it would be there in the first place, I don't want them to tell me, but no, I do so it can be treated and fixed.*

Try going to sleep with that running through your head! I was fine. I am fine. I did go to the doctor the next day, and it was an anxiety attack brought on by overthinking. It was actually triggered by my dad's good doctor report, oddly enough. He had called me to let me know about his checkup and told me the doctor said his ticker was great! That good news got me wondering how my ticker was, and so the spiral started. Ah, the power of suggestion!

Fear

Fear is one common overthinking trigger. In the above example, I got scared by a weird sensation and, having heart talk on my mind already, I freaked out. The negative thoughts started whirling, and I went through all three types of overthinking. I overgeneralized and applied the feeling to every heartbeat. After I monitored it, I went all-or-nothing. I was convinced that every peak and valley was extreme, I couldn't even register regular ones in my mind, and I knew I must be dying every split second in between. That was obviously catastrophic! I wasn't only failing *at life*, but my heart was failing *to live*. Clearly, fear misled me.

Perfectionism

Psychology Today describes perfectionism as life's "endless report card" (2022). How accurate is that? A healthy dose of perfectionism can be a good thing because it can motivate you to do your best and not settle for just good enough. For overthinkers, though, it can be a driving force to disaster.

Remember the two points at the beginning of this chapter? Overthinking begins as a helpful tool. Perfectionism does too. Your mind wants success. That's a good thing. However, if it continues past accomplishment, it may land on flawless insistence, and this is where it runs offtrack.

At this point, perfectionism stops you because, if you haven't landed on a solution that's good enough but you have to go with it, you go forward one step but then back two because it's not exactly right. *What if that solution doesn't work?* So you go over it again. Overthinking prevents you from trying something new because you worry that you won't get it right right away.

When I was an overthinker, it stunted my creativity. When I toyed with a creative project, I wouldn't get very far because my inner critic would speak up, tear it apart, rework every aspect, and stop me from doing it at all because it had me convinced it would never be perfect.

There's No Off Switch

This may sound more like a symptom than a cause. It's another chicken-or-egg perplexity. Do you overthink because your mental gears won't stop spinning, or is overthinking keeping those wheels turning? Either way, there's no off switch!

When you go to bed, your brain doesn't slide into park—or even neutral. It slips to overdrive. Instead of drifting off to dreamland feeling good about your day, your mind drifts like a NASCAR taking Turn 6 at Watkins Glen, and you find yourself completely off the restful track you aimed for. The best you can hope for is to run out of gas.

You Struggle to Make Decisions

This is another cause-or-effect question, and again, it can be either or both. If you have difficulty making decisions to begin with, you could end up spending inordinate amounts of time considering all outcomes. The opposite is also true: Considering all possible outcomes can keep your mind running and make it difficult, if not impossible, to land on one choice. If you're an overthinker, you likely spend a lot of time researching or seeking second opinions because you can't find satisfaction in your own solution. This leads to overanalyzing the new information, and the cycle continues.

BREAK THE CYCLE

While I was in the midst of the panic attack about my ticker flicker—the one triggered by my dad's positive health report—the anxiety kept driving my heart rate up and making it irregular. When I had a calm moment—an actual emotionally and mentally sound moment—nothing was out of the ordinary. But turning that switch on created potentially devastating physical effects on my body. It was crucial for me to seek help and find a solution, or my overall well-being would be compromised. It was time to break the cycle.

Overthinking is a habit. It's not a disease or disorder, and there are no medications to treat or cure it. Antianxiety drugs and antidepressants may lessen those accompanying symptoms, but they will do nothing to put the brakes on runaway thoughts. When overthinking becomes a problem in your life, you have to determine for yourself to take action to tame it.

Before we consider more aggressive approaches, let's take a look at how you can help yourself right now:

- **Squish the ANTs.** ANTs are automatic negative thoughts, which are a kind of cognitive distortion. They are spontaneous reactions to a trigger, usually a fear, a sense of danger, or something that fuels your anger. ANTs are learned responses that have become so practiced they occur as a reflex and are not carefully assessed. The first step to putting a stop to negative thoughts is to identify them.

Healthline suggests recording them in a journal. This way, you will recognize them when they pop up and actively shut them down before they spiral into overthinking. Here are some tips to get you started (Elmer, 2023):

○ First, write down the cause. Consider the four Ws: who, what, when, where.

○ Second, using only one word, describe your mood at the time of the trigger and note its intensity.

○ Third, write down what thoughts and images ran through your mind.

Review your notes to better understand what is triggering the negative thoughts and what you're telling yourself in response to them, and start thinking of ways you can change them.

- **Distract and redirect.** When you feel yourself going down the rabbit hole of rumination, change your focus. Do an activity you enjoy, one that involves brainpower and doesn't allow the mind to wander or continue to obsess. For example, try a new workout program. Make sure it's one you haven't done before so you have to pay attention to form and format. You could also volunteer with a cause you support. There's a horse ranch near my home that provides therapy to children with disabilities. When I was an overthinker, I volunteered there. It not only gave me a purposeful activity that kept my mind focused, but it also enabled me to bring joy to others and replaced my negative thoughts with positive ones.

- **See the big picture.** Consider this: Will the issues you're mulling over—and over and over and over—have any impact on your life 5–10 years down the road? So you had a typo on a slide in that client presentation. You won the account anyway! Will the client remember it later? In all likelihood, they've probably already forgotten, if they even noticed it at all. As the old saying goes, don't make mountains out of molehills.

- **Be nice to yourself.** This was a hard one for me. In fact, a good friend used to tell me frequently to stop being mean to me. At the time, I couldn't help it. It's a hazard of the habit. When I was an overthinker, I would get caught in the loop and end up solution-less and frustrated over having wasted so much time and energy on such insignificant matters, then I'd beat myself up for being so vulnerable to my thoughts and for letting them control me. My self-esteem would sink, my productivity would fail, and I had no one to blame but my own negative self-talk.

- **Don't be embarrassed to ask for help.** We're going to discuss several proven methods to overcome overthinking in the following chapters, but if, by the end of this book, you are still stuck in the cycle, please consider consulting a professional counselor. They may have more tools to help you change your mindset, find relief from your internal struggles, and arrive at a healthy state of well-being.

CHAPTER 2:

THE BENEFITS OF MINDFULNESS

Do not anticipate trouble or worry about what may never happen. Keep in the sunlight. –Benjamin Franklin

Mindfulness is an often-recommended practice that has proven to help overthinkers change their rumination habits. Having its roots in Buddhism, it has become a very beneficial exercise with applications not only in psychological spheres but also in physical health improvements as well.

WHAT IS MINDFULNESS?

Mindful's Susan Gillis Chapman says that mindfulness empowers us and keeps us from making matters worse (2019). It helps us remain steady. In essence, mindfulness is a state of awareness. It brings to your conscious attention what you are doing—spinning the wheels of your mind in perpetual analysis—and teaches you how to replace that tendency with actions to benefit your well-being. The key to its success is that it is a judgment-free zone. It is an activity you do for and by yourself, so there are no external critics. You must also not deem yourself inadequate in any way while performing these acts.

Keeping mindfulness judgment-free may be a challenge in itself, at least in the beginning. One major aspect of overthinking involves negative thoughts. Overthinkers tend to get frustrated with themselves for being unable to escape the rumination loop. They abuse themselves mentally and emotionally and beat themselves up internally. Mindfulness allows for none of that. It teaches that there is no right or wrong way to think or feel at any particular time. This frees you from believing yourself a failure and guides you along a path toward self-acceptance. When you practice mindfulness, you reside in the current moment. You focus on immediate sensations, and you don't fall back on past errors or project possible future derailments.

Mindfulness is the path you take to remove all of the negative voices that exist within you. It is the ability to be fully present in the moment. While you may not currently feel capable of doing that, the process is natural, and you already possess the instinctive skill. Mindfulness means maintaining control over not just your thoughts, which, as we've seen, can easily slip into repeat, but also over your feelings, surroundings, and physical sensations—anything that could trigger the cycle to start.

BENEFITS OF MINDFULNESS

As we discussed in the last chapter, overthinking is *not* problem-solving. It is actually counterproductive to that effort because it 1) creates more problems than it resolves, 2) drives up anxiety and deepens depression, 3) wastes energy that could have been used to put a plan into action, and 4) paralyzes your mind so you are unable to come to a conclusion. Mary-Beth Zolik of *EMDR Healing* tells us just how mindfulness practices stop the loop of repetition: "Mindfulness can help with this by placing an extra layer of awareness around our thinking, preventing us from being absorbed into our thoughts and giving us some detachment from them" (2020).

Dr. Jon Kabat-Zinn, a professor emeritus of medicine at the University of Massachusetts Medical School, developed the Mindfulness-Based Stress Reduction (MBSR) program in 1979 to introduce the Buddhist concept into American mainstream culture. According to the University of California Berkeley's *Greater Good Magazine*, thousands of studies have examined the practice over the past 40+ years, repeatedly documenting the positive aspects of mindfulness in general—and MBSR in particular—on the physical and mental health of people who practice it (*What Is Mindfulness?*, n.d.). The MBSR model has been adapted to suit hospitals, schools, veterans' centers, and prisons across the country, as well as innumerable therapeutic outlets and independent programs.

Kabat-Zinn explains that mindfulness is about systematically paying attention. You might say overthinking is systematic, and I suppose it is. Analyzing thoughts is certainly an organized process, but when the mind is unable to determine the conclusion of the matter, it ceases to be helpful. Kabat-Zinn's intent is to pay attention to the present moment with a methodical purpose. In a 2010 YouTube discussion with the Greater Good Science Center, he presents the analogy that we have only the present time to get our work done—office work, family work, relationship work—whatever you do to work at living. When we ruminate or overthink by incessantly trying to find a better way to, well, live, we squeeze out the present time until it is nearly nonexistent. However, Kabat-Zinn reminds us

The conditions are never actually right for being in the present moment, which is why we don't want to be there so much. But since it's never really satisfactory, we drive ourselves insane, really, trying to rearrange the deck chairs on the *Titanic* as opposed to sort of understanding that we are not the *Titanic* to begin with.

The present moment is fleeting as it is; overthinking wastes what little time you do have.

Scientific Evidence

Dr. Jon Kabat-Zinn developed his MBSR program at a scientific medical facility. He opened his Stress Reduction Clinic at the site, and by 1982, studies were already being done on the program's effectiveness. Initially devised to treat people with chronic pain and teach them meditation methods to relieve their discomfort, the concept quickly evolved into further-reaching health matters. Those who observed its effectiveness noticed how it not only relieved physical pain but it also lowered stress and reduced the impact of chronic illness.

Systemic research was later conducted by Richard Davidson of the University of Wisconsin at Madison. Davidson is one of the founders of the field of affective neuroscience, which combines the study of neuroscience with psychology to learn how the brain processes emotion, mood, and personality. Davidson's studies set up MBSR as the criterion by which research into mindfulness-based interventions is measured. Two separate clinical trials were conducted and their results were published in 2000 and 2008 in *The Journal of Consulting and Clinical Psychology*, which concluded that patients who underwent the MBSR program had 50% less chance of relapse from recurrent depression, and findings in *The Lancet* confirmed patients were successfully able to taper off medications due to the significant, long-term improvements they experienced by adhering to the MBSR system (Mindful Staff, 2022).

Mindfulness is now used to treat anxiety, depression, addiction, pain, obsessive-compulsive disorder (OCD), chronic illnesses, weight loss, and side effects of various medical treatments. The beauty is that anyone can put it into practice, from medical professionals to business leaders and professional athletes to the guy next door.

In the next section, we'll look at ways to apply the mindfulness approach in our lives. But first, let's consider just how the practice works on our minds and bodies to bring us that much-desired overall well-being (Mindful Staff, 2022):

- **Decreased anxiety and depression:** As mentioned before, science isn't sure which is the cause and which is the result, but experts in the field do agree that overthinking is correlated to both anxiety and depression. What relieves one area often benefits the other by default. Analysis of 47 studies determined that following a mindfulness program such as MBSR conclusively reduces the negative components of stress on the psyche. A review published in *JAMA Psychiatry* of 9 trials concluded that mindfulness-based cognitive therapy (MBCT) reduces the risk of relapse for up to 60 weeks, regardless of the patient's age, gender, education, or societal status, and was especially effective in people with initially high levels of depressive symptoms.

- **Improved mental clarity:** Analysis of 18 studies of 8-week MBSR and MBCT program participants showed improved cognition, including short- and long-term memory, self-awareness, and cognitive flexibility. Cognitive flexibility refers to being able to switch from one way of thinking to another or to redirect the mind from one task to another. In regard to overthinking, this has big implications because that's exactly what you need your brain to retrain itself to do. In a similar study, it was also shown to reduce the "attentional blink," or the time when new information is not received or recognized because the mind was too consumed with an existing thought or task.

- **Reduced mind wandering and overthinking:** As you reduce the attentional blink, you will become more aware of thoughts and opportunities you might otherwise have missed. Those subjects are no longer being overlooked while your brain runs circles about a past occurrence or future fret. Research published in the *Proceedings of the National Academy of Sciences* revealed that those who practice advanced mindful meditation experience less mind wandering and are able to put a stop to their ruminations more easily.

- **Boosted self-confidence:** A group of colleagues at the University of Westminster put a group of senior-level managers in the London area through a 12-week meditation program. Their results showed significantly improved self-confidence, moral intelligence, and vision sharing. It, however, did not enhance the individuals' position as role models or make them more likely to inspire their subordinates to take action in that brief observation period. It can be speculated, though, that as these individuals learn to display that newfound self-confidence, the subsequent effects will follow.

WAYS TO PRACTICE MINDFULNESS

When I was an overthinker, I thought about trying mindfulness practices. I read all about its origins, the many different methods, the benefits, and I got stuck in the analysis. *Does it really work? What if I miss a day? What happens when I stop doing it? Will I start overthinking again? What about this method… or that one… or this other one? Do they all generate the same results? Which is most effective? What if it's not?* Instead of choosing a technique and taking the first step, I thought through each step of one or the other activity and came to the catastrophized conclusion that debunked each step and determined none of them would ever work for me in any way.

I've got to tell you, just recalling this mind trap wears me out. When I was actually going through the experience, I was completely mentally and physically exhausted. I had definitely squeezed my present into oblivion, but I could not move forward until I had no energy left to entertain even one more trip around the overthinking loop. That's when I landed on the first technique we'll discuss below: mediation. It's actually where my mindfulness training began. I started there because it seemed to require the least effort from me. My brain was already overtaxed, so letting it rest and simply focus held great appeal. And thus began the first step of my recovery journey.

Mindfulness has branched out into many areas of interest, and people are constantly creating new and exciting ways to incorporate it into daily life. If you find that a traditional session isn't for you, try a different approach. Even if you run through several options, you haven't failed, because you have actively begun to pursue freedom from overthinking.

Meditation

At one time, meditation was thought of as a strange New Age concept that was steeped in Eastern philosophies. It was widely misunderstood, and therefore, mainstream Western culture was a bit suspicious of it. Defined by *Encyclopedia Britannica* as "private devotion or mental exercise encompassing various techniques of concentration, contemplation, and abstraction, regarded as conducive to heightened self-awareness, spiritual enlightenment, and physical and mental health," the technique has actually been practiced by nearly all known religions, including Roman Catholicism (Merkur, 2023). Though initially developed to help adherents dive deeper into their spirituality, throughout the 20th century, pop culture expanded it into something more versatile that could be applied to general well-being.

As meditation morphed from Hindu's yoga practices of body, mind, and soul purification to Chinese Buddhist and Japanese Zen interpretations, an unexpected trend in the 1960s made meditation vogue. The British rock sensation, the Beatles, had such a phenomenal following that it seems whatever they did was emulated everywhere. Their openly professed transcendental meditation (TM) practices became a huge commercial success throughout the decade, exporting Southern and Eastern Asian techniques to fans around the world as they searched inwardly for the source of self-love and love of others. As "peace, love, and rock and roll" rang out, so did the mantras of TM.

Let's get back to basics. Meditation is free thinking. It is not intended to solve problems or lay out careful plans. It has no room for judgment, and it has no predetermined destination. That doesn't mean your mind is an empty vacuum. Far from it! The intent of meditation is to explore and sense. In this realm, everything is momentous because you are probing the workings of your mind. It's all discovery as you focus intently on sensations, thoughts, and emotions by doing the following:

- **Put it on your schedule.** Set a specific time to meditate each day. Some people find it helpful to meditate as soon as they get up before life has the chance to distract them.

- **Find a comfortable place.** You need no special equipment, no meditation pillow or anything like that (unless you want one). Just sit somewhere comfortable that's free from interruptions, like cats, kids, or cell phones.

- **Close your eyes, relax your breathing, and lower your shoulders.** Prepare yourself to release your concerns and get ready to explore your inner world.

- **Observe the present moment.** There are many ways to do this, and we'll discuss some of them in later sections. For basic meditation, though, simply focus your mind on where you are right now, what's immediately around you, and what is in this little squeezed-out sliver of the present that you currently occupy.

- **Brush off judgments.** If you sense judgment rising, dismiss it. Now is not the time or place to analyze or criticize. Now is the time to observe and examine.

- **If your thoughts wander, rein them back into the present moment.** Sometimes being still and quiet can tempt our minds to roam, but following them is a different exercise. Right now, simply observe where they've wandered and bring them back in without reacting to them.

- **Be kind to yourself.** Remember this is a no-judgment zone. Don't criticize yourself for thinking of something peculiar. This is a time to adventure, and even odd thoughts are allowed. Just keep in mind that this is also not the time to analyze, so if something unusual pops into your mind, take note of it, let it go, and return to the present moment.

- **Ponder some fundamental elements.** Now that you're prepped and in position, consider these tips to keep your mind engaged and centered:

- Notice what your arms and legs are doing. Feel them. Are they tingly? Cold? Bent? Spend a few moments checking out their sensations.
- Notice your posture. Is it straight? Slouched? Is it comfortable? Readjust and observe anything new or different.
- If your eyes are open, what do you see? Shift your gaze. Do you see anything new? Do you see a familiar object from a new perspective?
- Feel your breath as it comes in and goes out. Is it deep or shallow? Does it speed up or slow down? Can you feel the air pass through your nose? The rise and fall of your chest?
- When you're ready, end the session. If your eyes are closed, flutter them open. Take one deep inhale and slow exhale, and then slowly stand up and move forward with your day.

Breathing Exercises

There are many types of mindful breathing exercises, but I like to begin with a yawn. That's right! A yawn. As I mentioned before, when I first started to experiment with mindful practices, I was utterly exhausted, body and soul. I yawned frequently, and as it turns out, I was engaging in a practice and didn't even know it.

Some people find it hard to relax or calm their minds when they've been in an active overthinking session. If you can't conjure up a real yawn, start with a fake one, and real ones will follow. This will move your focus from the thoughts in your mind to your physical bodily motions. When you yawn, observe the sensation. How did that brief pause feel? Yawn again, and this time incorporate a 20-second stretch. If you notice areas of tightness, try to relax them and yawn-stretch once more.

Now, you should be ready to set your intention on the present moment. Try this simple option to use your breath as an object of awareness:

- **Breathe slowly in and out.** Focus solely on each breath. Draw air deep into your lungs, inhaling through the nose. Release that slowly back out through your mouth, keeping your lips slightly parted. Pay attention only to the in and out of your breath.

- **Notice the location of each breath.** Is it in the nostrils right now? Has it settled in the lungs? By what path does it exit the body? At what placement did your chest rise and fall?

- **Take deeper breaths than normal.** Regular breaths are controlled by your autonomic nervous system, meaning you usually don't think about doing it. Your body does it involuntarily to keep you alive. However, we are able to manipulate breathing to an extent. Take a few regular breaths. How did that feel? Were they quick? Shallow? Did they have a certain rhythm? Now, slow that down. Pay attention to the speed of the breath and how deeply it fills your lungs. How was it different from a normal breath? Was the exhale different too?

- **Catch your breath.** If your mind wanders from the act of breathing to a new scent in the air or takes some other detour, again, rein it in and bring it back to the present moment. Focus once again on your breaths for a few moments longer, and then complete the session.

- **Make it fun.** Some people think simple breathing exercises are boring, so one way to make it interesting is to alternate nostrils. Just follow the steps above, but while plugging one nostril closed; repeat for the other side.

Five Senses Exercises

Another very common mindfulness exercise is to focus on each of the five senses. It's quick and requires very little time, so it can be done anytime or anywhere. If you find yourself stuck in the loop while waiting for a meeting to start, this is a good method to try.

By utilizing the five senses exercise, you can bring your awareness back to the current moment in a short amount of time. You need no special equipment, worksheets, or guidance recordings. Just notice things you are experiencing with each sense.

You can follow this order to practice the exercise. If you need to run through them again, or if you can't remember the order, simply switch it up:

- **Sight:** What five things can you see? Look around. Pick five things you wouldn't normally notice. Do you see that pattern in the concrete? Does the shape make you think of an animal? Look how worn the letters are on your keyboard. Does your dog have a unique pattern in its fur that you hadn't seen before? Give new attention to the details.

- **Touch:** What four things can you feel? Focus on four things you can touch. What do they feel like? Feeling the texture of your pants. Are they rough? Smooth? How does the sun feel on your skin? What about the flower petals in the vase on the table?

- **Sound:** What are three things you can hear? Listen carefully. Turn off your television or device. Hear the sounds all around you. Is a bird chirping outside? Did your child laugh? Did a car horn blare as it went by your window?

- **Scent:** What are two things you can smell? There's a reason popular air fresheners market to those of us who are "nose blind." We tend to filter out scents we frequently encounter. But now, it's time to zoom in on them, whether they're pleasant or unpleasant. Take a deep inhale when you open the bag of freshly ground coffee. Go back to those petals on the table and take in their aroma.

- **Taste:** What is one thing you can taste right now in this moment? Did you take a sip of the coffee you just brewed? How is it? Bitter? Smooth? Strong? Sweet? Or maybe you're chewing gum. Is it minty? Fruity? You could even draw air into your mouth and contemplate its taste.

Mindful Walking

So far, you've been still during your mindfulness practices, but you don't have to remain motionless to benefit from these activities. Here's a good one that gets you up and on the move while keeping an intentional awareness on the present moment: mindful walking.

Unlike the techniques listed so far, this one involves some physical exercise, although it doesn't have to be intense. You can begin by pacing the length of your hallway for a single minute. As you feel more comfortable, extend the time and distance to a walk around the block or eventually a hike through the park.

Like the yawn and five senses activities, mindful walking redirects your brain from your recurring thoughts to your bodily functions. It also incorporates some features from other practices. Be careful not to let your mind wander while you follow this advice:

- **Pay attention to each step.** Notice how each foot falls. Do you have a heavy step or a light one? Feel each part of your foot as it lands, bends, and lifts again. Can you sense the contraction of your leg muscles?

- **Count your steps while you breathe.** How many did you take during each inhale? Each exhale? Speed up or slow down and count again. Did the number change? Can you match your steps to your breaths?

- **Notice your lungs.** Don't force your breaths; just breathe normally. Do your lungs fill sufficiently? Do they struggle to hold air? Do they get shorter or longer as you adjust your stride?

- **Listen to the sounds around you.** If you're in your home, is music playing? If you're outdoors, are dogs barking? Did your heel crunch dry leaves? Is the wind whipping through the trees?

- **Appeal to your senses again.** Is the air cool or warm? How does it feel on your skin? Are there scents on the breeze? What are they? Flowers blooming in the park? Burgers grilling at the nearby restaurant? Is it sunset? What colors do you see in the sky?

- **Make it fun.** List something you see for every color of the rainbow. On longer walks, notice something that begins with each letter of the alphabet.

Coloring

This activity has gained popularity in recent years with the publication of many adult-oriented coloring books. Instead of simply drawn images of superheroes and ponies, these books feature very detailed drawings of things like mandalas, landscapes, and geometric forms. They're widely available in craft stores and hobby shops or online. If you're artistically inclined, you may even create your own artwork, sketches, or paintings. The purpose is, again, to shift the mind from internal overload to physical motion.

There aren't really any steps to follow for this technique, but here are some things that can help you stay in the present moment:

- **Choose your application.** Will you color with crayons, draw with pencils, sketch with markers, blend with charcoals, or paint with watercolors or oils? Will you use a canvas? A block of wood? Artist's paper? A coloring book? Choose only one per session.

- **Select an image or theme.** A good place to begin is with a prefabricated color-by-number product. This eliminates the possibility of getting caught up in overthinking because it reduces the number of options and colors available.

- **Apply color.** Focus on that one color. Is it bright? Soft? Light? Dark? Did you press down hard to leave the mark? How did your finger or hand feel?

When you change colors, notice how they contrast or complement each other. Stay focused on what's in front of your eyes and don't allow your mind to wander or speculate about the finished work.

- **Admire the completed image.** What feelings does it stir in you? Does it make you happy? Cheerful? Content? Satisfied?

- **Advance the exercise.** If you color for longer durations, try to incorporate breathing techniques into your actions.

Body Scan

This is a mindful practice I personally enjoy. I find it very relaxing despite being, at times, frustrating. I say it can be frustrating because if I begin when I am particularly stressed, sometimes an area I have already released will tense up again, and I will go back to the beginning to start over. You do not necessarily have to go back to the beginning, but my intent when practicing the body scan is to arrive at an overall place of peace. If one area remains out of balance, I focus on it some more.

Determine to be intentional and do the following:

- **Find a comfortable place away from distractions.** I prefer to lie down on a bed, sofa, or floor with my arms down by my sides.

- **Focus on one body part at a time.** Some suggest starting with your toes and working toward the top of your head, but I do the opposite. Again, mindfulness is a judgment-free zone with no right or wrong methodology. You choose what works best for you.

- **Close your eyes and take one deep inhale and slow exhale.** Envision the crown of your head and set your attention on how it feels right now. Is it tight? Does the scalp pull? Take a breath and let it out while releasing the tension from that spot. It may feel tingly or like a soft shower trickling down over your head.

- **Slowly progress from the top of your head.** Focus on one body part at a time. Include your ears, eyes, and mouth. Don't forget to cover both sides of the body. Because you have many body parts, this exercise may take some time, but that's okay. And, like me, you may need or want to start over if you feel yourself losing focus or tensing back up.

- **Wiggle your toes.** When you reach your feet, focus on each aspect from heel to toe. Notice physical sensations. Let your legs drop to the side if that's what they tend to do. As you finish the exercise, gently wiggle your toes to reawaken your body and flutter your eyes open. Remain in this relaxed state for a few moments before trying to stand so you don't get dizzy or fall.

- **Try an advanced technique.** To enhance the activity, imagine a color associated with the body part you are focusing on. For example, picture a yellow glow around your eyes and allow it to melt away tension in that area. Or if you sense pain in a certain body part, picture cool blue fading to warm lavender as you focus on and release it.

Journaling

Mindfulness is a journey. While its effects are profound and truly life-changing, it may take you a while to notice them. Not seeing immediate improvements can be discouraging. Keeping a mindfulness journal is a good way to track the changes you're making in yourself, and it gives you concrete proof that you are a work in progress.

Journaling allows you to focus your mind on one particular topic at a time. As you write out your thoughts, you transfer them from your mind to the paper (or computer), effectively breaking the overthinking cycle and allowing your brain to disengage. When you look back at your journal later on, you can reflect on those moments to see how you were able to finally shut them down and move forward.

While there is no right or wrong way to journal, there are a couple of different methods. Some people prefer to use a journal/planner to track not only the present moment but also prepare for upcoming events. If you are an overthinker who finds yourself worrying over the potential outcome of something that hasn't happened yet, this option may not be right for you. You should instead choose to journal just one day at a time. This will keep your focus on the immediate present and allow you to release the things affecting you right now.

Ryan Kane of *Mindfulness Box* offers a list of 59 prompts as well as a printable journal for those who need a boost to get started. Here are some suggestions to fill your first blank page (2022c):

- What do I feel at this moment? Do I feel good about myself? Am I happy? Am I upset? Am I content? How does my body feel physically in relation to these emotions? Is it calm? Relaxed? Jittery?

- Did anything make me smile today? What was it? How did I respond to that encounter? Did I communicate my joy to the source or person who contributed to it?

- Are there three things I am grateful for today? What are they? What do I appreciate about those things?

- Did any action come easily to me today? At work? At home? At play? What was it? Was it successful? How did it benefit me?

- What three things have caught my attention today? Are they things that have always been there that I just haven't noticed, or are they new to a place or setting? What made me notice them? What color(s) were they? Was I happy they were there?

- What three things do I like about where I live? Is it a quiet neighborhood? Are there many conveniences nearby? Do I feel safe here?
- What three things bring me joy? Can I access them more often? What about them pleases me?

Play With a Dog

Okay, this one's my favorite! Pets of all sorts can bring much joy and emotional comfort to their owners, but dogs have this unconditional love that they never hold back. It is commonly said that a dog is the only animal on the planet that loves you—its human—more than it loves itself. Dogs are not judgmental; they just want to comfort you and please you and make you happy. In this exercise, all you have to do is let them!

If you're lucky enough to have a pet—particularly a dog—try the following actions:

- **See your dog in the moment.** Notice how they approach each moment with curiosity, excitement, playfulness, and joy. See how they achieve present-moment awareness effortlessly without lingering on the past or fretting about the future.
- **Hug your dog.** Like some of the other techniques we've mentioned, hugging shifts the mind away from its swirling thoughts and onto the physical

sensation. You may have a very cuddly dog who hugs you back or one that just returns your hug with a slobbery kiss. Regardless, a big puppy hug will revive the mind-body connection and return your focus to the present.

- **Play.** Allow yourself to stop "adulting" for a moment and relieve your stress with a doggy romp. Play fetch, wrestle, dance, or play keep-away. Let the physical activity revive your mind and body in a moment of pleasure, a moment free from worry or concern and free from judgment.

- **Seek out a furry friend.** If you don't have a pet of your own, visit a friend who does or volunteer at a local shelter.

Author W.R. Purche once pointed out that all dog owners think they have the best, most loving, most loyal, most adorable dog on the planet. I know I do—wink-wink! In fact, when I was an overthinker, that was one thing I was certain of and never ruminated over or worried about.

I bet you believe your pooch is pretty great too. Guess what? According to Purche, we're both right! Research has proven that dogs make us happier and healthier. Owning a dog can reduce your risk of premature death by up to one-third, decrease loneliness by 40%, lower your blood pressure if you touch or talk to them, and increase your oxytocin levels, thus raising your "love hormone" levels and boosting your mood (Cohut, 2018; Pinkler, 2020; Donovan,

2016; Arford, 2020). Because they do not squeeze out their present by ruminating or overthinking, they remind us that it is indeed possible to focus on the here and now. When stressed out, play with your dog!

It Worked for Me

When I was an overthinker, one time I spent hours drafting an email to my boss asking for a promotion, only to delete it and never send it. Hours, I tell you! I would type my qualifications, include compliments from coworkers and clients, show how I would be the best candidate for the position, and then analyze the message: *That just sounds like I'm bragging. I'm exaggerating that part. My name was never on that project, so he has no way to confirm I did the work, and he'll think I'm making it up. Those praises came from the old boss who's no longer here; this guy won't care about that.* I was so worried about being rejected or seen as too pushy that I didn't take any action.

I later found out that my coworker, who had been in my same role but for only half the time, had been promoted. It was a wake-up call for me to start trusting myself and putting myself forward. I began to practice mindfulness techniques, first by doing basic breathing exercises and then progressing to body scans and journaling. This soon gave me the boost of self-esteem I needed to take small steps toward advocating for myself. I started with small requests, like asking for more responsibility on a project or requesting a meeting with my boss to discuss my career goals. With each success, my confidence grew, and I became more comfortable championing my skills and abilities.

As you can see, mindfulness worked for me! And it can work for you too. Each of the above practices can be varied by intensity and duration. While we have covered very basic techniques to get you started, remember that "the 'real' practice [of mindfulness] is living" (Meraji & Douglis, 2022).

CHAPTER 3:

COGNITIVE RESTRUCTURING

Nothing in life is more remarkable than the unnecessary
anxiety which we endure, and generally create ourselves.
–Benjamin Disraeli

Cognitive restructuring, also referred to as cognitive reframing, replaces irrational mental processes with logical ones. That sounds simple, but it is much easier said than done because, in overthinkers, those dysfunctional routines tend to become very deeply ingrained. Over time, they have become your automatic go-to responses. You've trained yourself for various "if this, then that" scenarios. When something comes up, you direct your thoughts to a particular route before considering the validity of your assessment. Actually, if you are an overthinker, you may not be able to properly assess the soundness of your determination to begin with. You've gotten caught in the overanalysis loop so often that instead of assessing a response, you skip it altogether and default to a distorted position.

Remember that overthinking is a habit, and with diligent work, habits can be broken. In this chapter, we will gain a better understanding of why cognitive distortions are so readily accepted by our minds, why we embrace these dysfunctional thoughts as legitimate resolutions, and most importantly, how we can re-establish functional thought systems.

Before we dive into cognitive restructuring, though, we need to take a look at the psychotherapeutic practice it is associated with: cognitive behavioral therapy (CBT). The goal of CBT is to identify ineffective thoughts, behaviors, and emotional responses and replace them with more positive and productive ones. In doing so, it combines cognitive strategies with behavioral approaches to bring about improved mental well-being and stability.

WHAT IS COGNITIVE BEHAVIORAL THERAPY?

Dr. Aaron T. Beck developed cognitive behavioral therapy (CBT) in the 1960s when trying to prove current psychoanalysis theories invalid. His studies revealed a strong correlation of erroneous thinking to psychological symptoms and conditions like depression, anxiety, and obsessive-compulsive disorder (OCD) and led him to conclude "that dysfunctional thinking was behind all psychological disturbances" (Sutton, 2017). He determined not to let that realization drop and came up with a treatment that transformed modern psychotherapy.

Beck's premise centered on three views: that hidden thought processes are occurring in the mind, that these processes influence our emotions and behaviors, and (the good news) that we *can* alter these processes.

Distorted Cognition and Dysfunctional Thinking

Cognitive distortion is faulty thinking. It involves biased responses to the world around us. These are usually subtle thoughts that appear to be nonthreatening and are easily accepted into our beliefs. Because we do not recognize them as errant, we reinforce them and unconsciously make them part of our daily repertoire.

For overthinkers, this can spell disaster. All distorted thought is inaccurate. We may not sense immediate harm, but when embraced, these dysfunctional ideals lead to blatantly false beliefs that can result in psychological damage. People who struggle with depression are particularly vulnerable to the ill effects of distorted thinking because they develop a dependency on what they perceive to be the truth in their negative self-thoughts. They confine their own minds in a prison of their own making, believing they're not good enough and committing themselves to self-despair. Again, experts are uncertain which is the cause and which is the effect, but cognitive distortion and depression have been proven to go hand in hand (Ackerman, 2017).

We touched on this subject in the first chapter when we talked about three of the most common cognitive distortions: overgeneralizing, all-or-nothing thinking, and catastrophizing. But there are several other forms, including the following (Ackerman, 2017):

- **Discounting positive experiences:** Whereas overgeneralization and catastrophizing focus on negatives and convince you those are the only destined outcomes, discounting the positive actually acknowledges positives but dismisses them and attributes them to some other coincidence or occurrence. This action prevents you from receiving compliments or commendations because you convince yourself that the good outcome was mere happenstance, and you continue to feed your negative self-talk. **Minimizing** is a similar occurrence in that it discounts the significance of an important achievement. For example, a star athlete may dismiss their record-setting performance and believe they're just a mediocre player.

- **Accepting emotions as fact:** This sort of response is often seen in alcoholics and drug abusers. When their minds are manipulated by a substance, they incorrectly interpret events and convince themselves the situation is real and valid. They might convince themselves that their partner is unfaithful and continue in that belief when sober, even though it is founded in falsehood.

- **Making predictions based on no tangible evidence:** Commonly referred to as fortune-telling—and I don't mean the prognosticating sort—this misthought is similar to all-or-nothing thinking. In this case, you predict a future occurrence based on one unsupported idea. For example, a friend might say they will never find love because they have not found it yet. Nothing concrete substantiates the conclusion.

- **Believing you know what someone else is thinking:** Mind reading occurs when you're so sure you know how another person will respond to you that you emotionally paralyze yourself. This habit is both presumptuous and devastating.

When I was an overthinker, this was a particularly bad habit of mine. And let me tell you, you don't need to know the other person in real life. This dysfunctional thinking can apply to virtual friendships on social media as well. One time, I shared a reel on Instagram and a follower replied by direct message. I was excited but didn't respond right away. I saw it and sat there and thought about it. I wrote a response and then reread it. *I shouldn't include that emoji. They're going to think it's juvenile.* Revised and reread. *No! They're going to doubt I really have this experience and think I don't have any authority to talk about this subject like this.* Revised and reread. *I'll put that emoji back. They'll think it looks friendly, and I'll seem more relatable.* Revised and reread. *Oh, that's too many exclamation points! They'll think I'm yelling at them.* In the end, I just clicked thumbs-up to like the message without corresponding at all.

This also involves a little bit of transference because our negative self-talk has us convinced that the other party will judge us in the same manner we judge ourselves. *If I'm thinking those doubts and criticisms about my own posts, others must be too.* You can end up catastrophizing the whole communication process. *Awkward.*

- **Taking everything personally:** A very close friend of mine does this. I unintentionally hurt their feelings numerous times until I realized they internalized every negative word about any situation in which they were involved. Though my words were about general situations, if my friend was present or participated in any way, they felt I was aiming my discontent directly at them. This distortion is detrimental to relationships because the person who takes it all personally is often offended by their friends and loved ones, and their friends and loved ones find themselves walking on eggshells to avoid inflicting that injury.

- **Making "should" statements:** We've all bought into this one before! You know you've said it too: "could've, would've, should've." This is a very common overthinking loop. It occurs when we get stuck on a past event that didn't work out the way we hoped it would, and we spin our mental wheels considering how things *would have* been better if only we *could have* done this and, wow, we *should have* done that.

When you participate in CBT, you learn to evaluate your thought processes more realistically. With guidance and practice, you identify which automatic thoughts are maladaptive—which ones make you embrace negative thoughts and behaviors and make you avoid new experiences—and you work your way toward trustworthy introspection.

WHAT IS COGNITIVE RESTRUCTURING?

As we live our lives and encounter new experiences, we create some shortcuts in our thought patterns. We make certain presumptions and establish ways of responding to circumstances, then we stash them away in little file cabinets in our minds. This way, we don't have to reinvent the wheel every time we come across those events again; we just pull the file. The problem, as we've seen, is that those methods are not always reliable.

When cognition becomes self-defeating and thought patterns lead to destruction, we must find ways to redirect them. Let's take a look at some of the best ways to realign faulty perspectives by reframing them with evidence-backed, unbiased, non-skewed, accurate beliefs.

Many people choose to partner with a therapist, but most of the following techniques can move you toward a healthier mindset on your own (Stanborough, 2020; Ackerman, 2018):

- **Asking "What if?" or "So what?":** I like this one! On the surface, it seems a little uncaring. *What if that does happen? So what?* But let's listen to that in a different tone: *What will really happen if this particular scenario plays out? What will you do—what real actions will you take—in that case?* Do you hear the appeal to logic in the second version? What often happens with overthinking is that we go to the worst-case scenario. You've already seen that in overgeneralizing, all-or-nothing thinking, and catastrophizing. This technique involves your making two lists: a glass-half-empty one and a glass-half-full one. For each dysfunctional thought you encounter, consider a negative outcome (half-empty) and a positive one (half-full) and write down "What if?" or "So what?" if that happens for each possibility. This will help you see that you could and would carry forward no matter what happened, and it will reshape that errant thought. When I was an overthinker, I was always anxious about conflicts with my coworkers. One time during a project meeting, my colleague Sarah suggested an idea that I didn't agree with. I automatically went to the futile what-ifs and so-whats: *This is no good. What if it tanks? Will the boss fire us? Will the client reject it? Will the client never work with us again? Will the boss blame me even though it was a collaborative effort? Will Sarah blame me and take credit for anything that doesn't fail herself? What will happen if I say nothing?*

Well, I was so worried about creating friction that I said nothing and went along with it. The idea turned out to be a disaster, and our team missed an important deadline. My boss was furious and, yes, he did blame me for not speaking up. I realized then that by avoiding conflict, I was actually hurting myself and my team. I learned from the experience to ask the productive questions of *What will really happen if this particular scenario plays out? What will you do—what real actions will you take—in that case?* And from that point on, I made a conscious effort to voice my concerns, even if they opposed the ideas of my coworkers. I found that by respectfully expressing my opinion, we were able to come up with better solutions together.

- **Gathering evidence:** You can't break or change a habit until you know the error you're making, and you can't identify that without tracking the triggers. Does a particular person seem to be present each time? Does it happen when you've been to a certain place? Did the event spark a memory? Is a specific atmosphere common to the start of your overthinking? For example, does it frequently happen when you must speak at a board meeting? The next section carries this concept further and provides a worksheet outline for you to record daily evidence.

- **Generating alternatives:** If mind reading is one of your cognitive distortions—if you *know* what the other person will think and generate your response as a reaction to that—this technique is for you. Instead of predetermining someone else's cognition, consider some alternatives. For example, don't jump to the conclusion that your coworkers were talking about you because they got silent when you entered the room. Instead, consider other possibilities, like their conversation naturally ran to its conclusion, they weren't really conversing but were merely passing the salt, or some other situation, and you may realize that you didn't *know* their minds so well after all.

- **Questioning by the Socratic method:** Socrates, the Greek philosopher who was sentenced to death in 399 B.C.E. for corrupting the Athenian youth with his ideology, is considered the founder of Western philosophy. Though he left no written works behind, his students—most famously Plato—recorded their interactions in question-and-answer conversation format. I myself ascribe to this technique and am a big proponent of asking questions. How else do you learn? How else do you solve challenges? How else do you get what you're after? By Socratic questioning, the teacher does not simply fill the student's mind with information, but both teacher and student work together to discover knowledge. The following are some questions to pose to yourself regarding your distorted cognition:

- o Is what I'm overthinking realistic?
- o Is this thought based on facts or feelings?
- o Is there evidence to validate this thought?
- o Is the evidence accurate, or am I misinterpreting it?

- **Using guided imagery:** Guided imagery is a visualization technique in which you focus on pleasant images. By doing so, you replace the negative thoughts and feelings you were previously entrenched in and shift your intent to something positive. This technique is, as the name suggests, guided by a therapist and can be utilized during an in-office session or by playing a scripted recording during a time you establish on your own.

Keeping a Thought Log

When I was an overthinker, this practice helped me make tremendous progress. It takes the mindfulness journal and builds on it. In your mindfulness journal, you recorded the thoughts you were contemplating in the present moment. This helped to break the overthinking cycle by giving rumination action. It got you out of your mind and into bodily movement. It disengaged your brain and gave you a reference book to look back on the things that consumed your mind, the feelings you associated with those things, and the behaviors that resulted. The thought log provides deeper analysis and, in the end, a confirmation record that you *can* do these things, you *can* break the cycle, and you *can* reach a healthy mental state.

Courtney Ackerman of *Positive Psychology* provides some thought log suggestions (2017):

- Create a worksheet with six columns. You can draw it on paper or utilize your computer software or an app. Label the columns as follows: date/time, occurrence, ANTs, associated emotion(s), initial response, more beneficial response.

- Recall a recent event about which you overthought and fill in the table you just created.

- In the "ANTs" column, write down how much you believed—or how convinced you were of—the faulty thoughts.

- In the "response" column, note which cognitive distortions you were displaying and why they were errant. Write down your worst-case scenario. How likely did you think that was to occur?

- In the "more beneficial response" column, write down adaptive thoughts to counter the dysfunctional ones. Consider a best-case scenario. How likely do you think that would be to occur if you responded with valid cognition?

- When the worksheet is complete, review it to see if you still believe your distorted perceptions as much or whether challenging them helped you to see their inaccuracy.

- Do you feel differently now than you did at the beginning of the exercise?

Collect these experiences each time you find yourself caught in the overthinking cycle. Over time, you will build yourself an arsenal of proof, a treasure bin from which you can pull confident moments. As you look back on these times, you will gradually see the errors of your former thoughts more clearly, and you'll actually become disgusted by them. You'll be surprised that you were so deceived, but you won't wallow in negative self-talk because you will have learned that those were deceptions—they weren't your true beliefs—and you will find strength and determination to keep moving ahead because you'll find confidence in how you overcame them. Then, you will more quickly and more readily shun errancy and accept valid truth. *That* is becoming your new go-to as you trek slowly but surely toward a brighter future.

CHAPTER 4:

BUILDING RESILIENCE

It has been well said that our anxiety does not empty tomorrow
of its sorrows, but only empties today of its strength.
–Charles Spurgeon

Resilience is a physics term. It refers to the ability of a "strained body" that is under "compressive stress" to regain its shape and restore its size (Merriam-Webster, n.d.-f). Are you a strained body under compressive stress? You may not literally be in a state of contortion, but your mind can certainly feel that way during and after a time of rumination.

How well do you cope, adapt, and survive in this world under the duress of overthinking? How quickly do you return to form? Do you bounce right back after getting caught in a thought loop, or do you linger awhile in a pit of self-abuse and negative self-talk? Developing resilience will help you navigate not only the hazards of modern society but also the distorted cognitions and destructive contemplations that repeatedly run through your mind.

WHAT IS RESILIENCE?

The more general definition of resilience describes an object's—or a person's—ability to recover from change. In psychological circles, we can define it by how well we cope with difficult situations in life. Most often, we think of trauma or stress, but an event doesn't have to be a physical occurrence for it to affect your mental state and impact how well you recover. An adverse incident can be any sort of disturbance that upsets your normal balance and leads you to an unexpected response or reaction.

"Normal." I shouldn't have used that word! Who defines what normal is anyway? When I was an overthinker, I often spun my mind in circles over that word. The thing is, it never had to do with *my* normal but always had to do with what other people—and society in general—said normal should be. I have since learned a much better way to understand this concept: homeostasis.

Homeostasis occurs when you're in a state of equilibrium. Biologically, it refers to an organism's ability to sustain health. In other words, it's your body's way of maintaining a steady temperature, blood sugar, weight, sleep, hunger, and other physiological functions. Homeostasis is like a checks-and-balances system that monitors and maintains your internal state. It also sustains your mental condition.

Emotional homeostasis refers to "emotional stability in the face of uncertainty," according to Patrick Williams and Howard Nussbaum of the University of Chicago (2016). They describe it as part of the affective dimension in Monika Ardelt's Three-Dimensional Wisdom Scale. In the affective dimension, you display sympathetic and compassionate love for others. In this realm, you not only feel positive emotions and exhibit positive behaviors toward others, but you also have an absence of indifference and negativity toward others (Macdonald, n.d.).

To put it simply, you are emotionally and intellectually balanced. I would consider that the foundation of "normal," wouldn't you?

Back to resilience. Homeostasis is hard to retain. Any number of conflicts, both internal and external, can throw things off balance. In homeostasis, we experience positive emotions; in survival mode, we experience negative ones. However, survival mode is designed by nature to return us to homeostasis. John Montgomery of *Psychology Today* tells us "Every type of negative emotion that we experience… help[s] motivate behavior that will bring us back into homeostasis. Homeostasis is where our bodies and brains want us to be whenever possible" (2012).

For example, a physical injury can upset physiological structure and throw emotions out of whack. You may find yourself ruminating about what caused the injury, how you could have avoided it, what will happen as you heal, how you will overcome the impairment, if it will affect you long-term, what the physical scar will look like, what the emotional scar will feel like, and many other things. To halt these thoughts and return to homeostasis, you must develop resilience.

The good thing is that this drive for balance occurs almost automatically. Your mind and body want to be stable, both emotionally and physically. Developing resilience will help you know how to respond to the difficult events you face without distorting your response. Resilience can reduce feelings of anxiety and depression, and it can lessen your likelihood of developing more serious mental health conditions by offsetting the effect trauma and crisis have on you. You will be better able to handle and overcome challenges.

The Mayo Clinic suggests the following activities in order to help you increase resilience (2022b):

- **Connect to your network.** Establish strong, healthy relationships with family members, friends, and others in your community who will support and encourage you through good times and bad. You might consider volunteering with or joining a faith-based or spiritual organization.

- **Give each day meaning.** Each day, make it your intention to do something of significance. It doesn't have to be big! Just set daily goals that give each moment purpose.

- **Don't reinvent the wheel.** Learn from your past, both the mistakes and the successes. You're still here, so clearly you survived the bad times. And I'm sure the successes didn't come easily, so there are bound to be moments when you had to persevere and work hard to achieve those accomplishments. Remind yourself of them.

- **Don't wish; act.** Your situation can improve, but you have to work at it. It won't just happen on its own.

- **Tend to your needs.** Take up hobbies you enjoy. Go new places and see new things. Eat healthy food, participate in physical activity, practice mindfulness, and make sure you are the best you that you can be.

- **Stay hopeful!** You can't change the past no matter how much you overthink those old conversations and events, but the future is wide open, and the present is the ideal place to begin. As Aristotle once said, "Hope is a waking dream" (n.d.).

Apply these concepts in your life. Your homeostasis will be restored, and you will be able to take on the world with confidence and resilience.

Emotions

Emotions can make you say "Oof!" Though there are only six basic ones, the shades and variations of those six are so vast that they complete a sort of color wheel. They can be mild or intense. They can appear suddenly or steal in slowly, but whether they sneak up or bear down, it seems we never experience a moment free from emotion.

Ekman's Six Basic Emotions

Dr. Paul Ekman, the famed psychologist who co-discovered micro emotions, established through his intense studies across international cultures six universal emotions that are inherent to all people (Cherry, 2022):

- **Anger:** Often considered negative, this very powerful emotion can be a good thing when it triggers you to make changes to situations that are harmful. Frustration, aggravation, and irritability fill this category, which is pretty easily identified by frowns, scowls, and downcast eyebrows as well as a loud, rough voice and occasional aggression.

- **Disgust:** Anything you perceive as unpleasant can result in a feeling of disgust. It could be a noxious odor like rotten garbage or graphic violence depicted in a film. You might plug your nose, gag, or turn away.

- **Fear:** Being scared is meant to be helpful. It kick-starts the fight-or-flight response to move us out of harm's way. If, however, it triggers an over-sensibility to imagined threats, it can create anxiety, increase our heartbeat, and literally take our breath away.

- **Sadness:** Being sorrowful is common. We often find ourselves upset when things don't go as planned. Grief, disappointment, and hopelessness commonly accompany frowning, crying, and withdrawal from those we're close to. Depression can result from extended periods of sadness.

- **Surprise:** Surprises can be good and bad. A surprise birthday party can be a fun, positive surprise, but someone jumping out at you with a weapon is not just negative but also absolutely terrifying. When you are surprised, you might scream or gasp, raise your eyebrows, or jump.

- **Happiness:** Joy is unequivocally a pleasant state. It is often sought, and many books have been written about its pursuit. Signs of happiness are smiles, laughter, and contentment. You'll have a sense of well-being and may display that with a relaxed posture and cheerful voice.

As time progressed, Ekman further developed his list to include more complex emotions, like excitement, pride, and embarrassment. His initial six are considered primary emotions, those that are the body's first response to a stimulus. Secondary emotions are natural extensions of the basics. They are often learned and habitual and can be errant—much like distorted cognitions. For example, instead of feeling fear, you may feel resentment toward the cause of the fear. Your personal experiences and influences from those around you can affect the intensity, variation, and degree of emotion you sense.

SELF-COMPASSION

Where does compassion fit in? Compassion is an extension of happiness. It may be triggered by a negative emotion like anger or disgust because it involves taking on someone else's pain and taking action to relieve it. Compassion takes empathy and puts it to work.

Compassion implies an outward expression of the sympathy you feel toward someone who's struggling. The term self-compassion is easy to break down, but its literal sense sounds strange: to suffer together with yourself. When you turn compassion inward and apply it to yourself, you acknowledge the connectedness of humanity and realize you are one with the many. You understand the need for people to feel for each other and to extend kindness and aid without withholding it for judgment or cruelty. You reach out to others to soften distress, not to pity or simply feel bad about their situation. Likewise, you can reach inward to relieve your own affliction with gentle benevolence. It shows that you care about yourself and your own well-being.

Christopher Bergland of *Psychology Today* explains that there are three components of self-compassion (2020). Kristen Neff, cofounder of the *Center for Mindful Self-Compassion*, further expounds on those concepts, as discussed below (2020):

- The first component is the ability to be kind to yourself, forgive your mistakes, and criticize yourself less often. It involves showing yourself warmth and understanding rather than judgment and insult. We are all human. We will fail sometimes. No one can live life exactly to their standards. When those moments of what you deem inadequacy occur, don't ignore them but also don't berate yourself for not achieving the success you'd hoped for. Allow yourself room to mess up. Know that errors are inevitable, but don't default to those old dysfunctional thoughts. Focus instead on the positives, the good things you did achieve, and move forward with encouragement.

- The second component is to recognize that the basic primary emotion of happiness is inherently intermingled with pain, struggle, and challenge. Being human means you are vulnerable, and suffering and imperfection are part of the shared human experience. You are not alone in your experiences.

- The third component is to be consciously aware of unpleasantries in each moment but not let them consume you. Don't suppress negative emotions just because you don't like them; similarly, don't exaggerate them or allow them to overwhelm you. Remember that homeostasis we talked about earlier? Apply it here. Find the equilibrium. Acknowledge your pain and put empathy into action to bring about relief without overidentifying with negative reactivity.

Some people worry that putting so much effort into their own self-awareness will leave them consumed with themselves to the neglect of other relationships. This is not true! In fact, self-kindness, self-care, and self-empathy do not equal selfishness or narcissism. Kristen Neff tells us that "Research indicates that in comparison to self-esteem, self-compassion is associated with greater emotional resilience, more accurate self-concepts, more caring relationship behavior, as well as less narcissism and reactive anger" (*Self-Compassion vs. Self-Esteem*, 2016). As you work on those aspects of self, you will develop greater self-esteem, increase your self-confidence, and expand your compassion for yourself and others.

Self-compassion is not based on any personal assessment. It's not about your value, and it's not about how good you feel. It's about being kind to yourself, acknowledging your struggles and your weaknesses without judgment or condemnation, and allowing yourself to be human. It's not about hiding anything or impressing other people. It's all internal. It's all *you* treating yourself well.

Self-Esteem

Self-esteem, in contrast to self-compassion, does have to do with our sense of self-worth. Do we think we contribute great value to society? Do we have a long list of achievements to confirm this? Those who struggle to maintain healthy self-esteem often compare themselves to others in order to prove that they stand out from the crowd and are special. They try to let their awards fill the emptiness inside with significance. Sometimes, they conceal their vulnerabilities in order to keep up the facade that they believe in their own importance, and they may put others down just to feel better about themselves. Do you find these tendencies in yourself? Unhealthy self-esteem can give you a false sense of pride and threaten relationships. It can easily lead to overthinking because you're constantly assessing and reassessing your value.

On the other hand, those with healthy self-esteem are confident in their abilities. They don't fear failure because their setbacks don't define them. They don't compare themselves to other people or to their own past because they accept their unique contribution to society, family, community, and life in general.

There is a caveat, though: Self-esteem is unstable. A high point may not last. Self-esteem can fluctuate with the tides of your emotions and experiences. Our goal in this section is to help you learn how to level it back out, allow it to boost your self-confidence, and use both to enhance your self-compassion as you work to build resilience.

The Mayo Clinic suggests the following ways to improve self-esteem based on both cognitive behavioral therapy and acceptance and commitment therapy (2022):

- **Know your triggers.** Recognize situations that deflate your self-esteem. Perhaps a work presentation didn't go as well as planned, and now you feel unworthy of your position or level of responsibility. Maybe you had a disagreement with your spouse and now you doubt their commitment or the sureness of your relationship. When you become aware of what sets the drop in motion, you can take preventative steps to maintain it.

- **Notice your thoughts about your triggers.** What do you tell yourself about these situations? How do you interpret them and their effects on you? Are your thoughts positive, negative, or neutral? Are they rational or irrational? Is there evidence to support your beliefs about the event? Would you express these thoughts verbally to a friend? If you wouldn't speak these things to another person, then don't tell them to yourself.

- **Put negative thoughts to the test.** Rarely is there only one way to view a situation. Is your view backed by facts and logic? Is there a different explanation? Challenge your thoughts, even if your belief is long-held. Just because it's the way you've always assessed things doesn't mean it's the right or best perspective to take. Try to avoid all-or-nothing thinking in which you interpret things as either entirely good or entirely bad. Balance your analysis. Also, don't dwell solely on the negatives. Remember the good that came from the situation and build yourself up by focusing on what went right. And be careful not to turn those positives into negatives.

- **Make adjustments where necessary.** Replace negative thoughts with positive ones. Forgive yourself for any mistakes you made. Don't "could've, would've, should've" things. You can't change what happened with if-onlys. Learn from the experience as a whole, including both the positive and the negative aspects. Let negative thoughts prompt you to try more productive, healthier habits. Encourage yourself; don't discourage yourself. Perhaps it wasn't a total success, but it wasn't a complete disaster either.

- This may sound odd, but repeat your negative thoughts. Restate them several times. You will begin to hear how automatic and inaccurate they are, and it will help you realize they have no significance, that they are just empty words.

- Allow yourself to feel your negative thoughts. Accept that you experienced them but don't be overwhelmed. It doesn't mean you have to like them, but if you acknowledge them in this way, you will lessen the power they hold on your responses and behavior.

Some of these steps may seem counterintuitive, but as you go through them, you will change the way you think. You'll be less prone to drops in self-esteem, and you will accept your personal value. As your self-esteem increases, so will your self-confidence and your emotional well-being.

Self-Confidence

Self-confidence means trusting yourself to be able to complete a task. It means you know you have the ability to take on a project and do it well. You are certain that you're capable of completing it without fail. You believe in your aptitude and are self-assured.

When I was an overthinker, I struggled with this. I knew I had aptitude and abilities. Having reached the level of success I did in the corporate world reinforced those faculties. But when it came to application, the wheels of my mind spun out of control with doubt. It didn't matter what accomplishments appeared beside my name, whenever a new opportunity arose, my overthinking shredded any confidence I had in my competence.

Battered self-confidence can have a sinking effect on job performance, academics, and relationships. Because you perceive yourself to lack the ability to succeed in these areas, others will follow your lead and show little confidence in you too. However, if you boost your confidence, you will also boost the control you have over your life, find more success in your personal life and in your professional life, and enhance your overall well-being.

Here are some simple things you can do to grow your self-confidence:

- **Put effort into your wardrobe and appearance.** Practice daily hygiene, dress in clean, wrinkle-free clothing, and make yourself presentable to the world. You will feel good about yourself when you are put together.

- **Exercise regularly.** You don't have to be a gym rat, but you should get at least 30 minutes of cardio exercise 3 times a week. It will strengthen your heart, lungs, and muscles, and it will also improve mental clarity and potency.

- **Assess and pursue your strengths.** What are you good at? What comes easily to you? What have you found success doing? Take note of these things and seek out ways to utilize them in your work, hobbies, and daily living.

- **Be thankful.** Notice the good. Express gratitude for what you have, for your home, your loved ones, your career, and whatever brings you joy and contentment.

- **Don't compare yourself to others.** A popular maxim advises that the only person you should compare yourself to is yourself: Strive to be a better you today than you were yesterday.

- **Set small goals.** As you achieve those, incrementally make them longer-term and more challenging to accomplish. This way, you will build on your successes.

- **Surround yourself with a solid support system.** Having friends and loved ones on your side will encourage you to see the good in yourself and help you gain the boost you need when your internal support system struggles.

Having self-confidence brings nothing but perks. It improves your performance at work, school, athletics, hobbies… in whatever you find yourself doing. It improves relationships because you will find faith in yourself and your own contributions to them, and you will have the courage to take steps to improve them—or to walk away from unhealthy situations. It will also make you more resilient because you will not only know of your capabilities, but you will also trust in them, and you will believe you can bounce back from challenges.

Self-Compassion Dos and Don'ts

On your journey to improve your self-compassion, give yourself an advantage and keep the following dos and don'ts in mind:

Do:

- Treat yourself and others with respect.
- Appreciate your uniqueness.
- Talk about your struggles.
- Consider consequences before responding or reacting.
- Consider alternative solutions.
- Focus on your strengths.
- Stay focused on solutions.

Don't:

- Critique or judge yourself harshly.
- Compare yourself to others.
- Isolate yourself because you think you don't fit in.
- Punish yourself.
- Lock yourself in an emotional prison of your own perspective.
- Go to extremes (all-or-nothing, catastrophizing).
- Shame yourself for mistakes.

SELF-COMPASSION EXERCISES

To reiterate, self-compassion is putting empathy into action in regard to your own well-being. A lot of people struggle in this area. They're great at expressing compassion for others. They often step up to help others out of difficult situations or to improve someone else's condition, but they neglect themselves. Do any of the following examples describe you?

- You berate yourself for the aspects you messed up instead of congratulating yourself for a job well done.
- You appreciate someone else's good work but overlook your own accomplishments.
- You smother yourself in guilt and shame when you make a mistake.

- You give in to feelings of frustration and overwhelm instead of embracing a challenge and finding a solution.
- You fall into "could've, would've, should've" thoughts and beat yourself up over something you "should've" done differently.
- You reprimand yourself for repeating a mistake.
- You criticize yourself for being indecisive.

When you practice self-compassion, you give yourself the same benevolence you give to others. Tchiki Davis of *Psychology Today* suggests doing the following activities to develop more self-compassion and boost your self-love (2021):

- **Write a letter to yourself.** Imagine that you are someone you know who is in need of kindness. Now, write a caring word to that person. When done, read it aloud to yourself. This exercise can decrease depression and increase joy.
- **Release negativity.** Next time you find yourself consumed with negative thoughts, picture fluffy clouds in a blue sky. Assign each negative thought to a cloud and watch it blow away. This exercise can help you let go of negativity and know it may be replaced with positivity.
- **Stand up to your self-bully.** Taking a lot of harsh judgment from your inner critic? Stand up for yourself! Why are you telling yourself these

negative things and treating yourself so poorly? Question your bully's motivation and fight against self-critical thoughts.

- **Forgive yourself.** It's okay to make mistakes; it's not okay to beat yourself up over them. You can't change the past or correct errors you've already made. Apologize to yourself if necessary and move on to an emotionally healthier, happier future.

When you have resilience, you harness your inner strength—that comes from your self-compassion, self-esteem, and self-confidence—to battle the challenges you face. You are certain that *you do possess the abilities* to tackle the situation, you rely on the knowledge that *you are able to do this*, and you pull from experience that affirms you've been able to handle it previously and *you can do it again*. Resilience doesn't eliminate problems, but it will help you prevent them from pushing you into overthinking overdrive.

CHAPTER 5:

PROBLEM-SOLVING STRATEGIES

Take time to deliberate, but when the time for action has arrived, stop thinking and go in. –Napoleon Bonaparte

Some people believe the more they think on a topic, the more likely they are to arrive at the best solution—or to at least keep a bad decision from turning out disastrous. But as psychotherapist Amy Morin explains, continuously thinking about a problem will not bring about its solution (2019). Overthinking increases stress, but Morin points out a key affirmation that you are genuinely solving a problem: Your stress—anxiety, worry, depression, and physical symptoms they've brought along, like headaches, muscle aches, fatigue, and stomach discomfort—will instead lessen.

I don't know about you, but I audibly said, "Ahhh," in relief.

If you're still certain you're problem-solving and not overthinking, ask yourself the following questions:

- **Is the solution to the problem in my hands?** *You* cannot solve some problems. As we discussed before, some problems are beyond your power, like a failed economy. (Remember? *You* can't solve all the world's problems.) Or perhaps you're trying to fix a mistake you made in the past, and because it's over and done, it cannot be changed. You can, however, respond differently to similar situations in the future. Altering your emotional response might be *the solution* to the problem at hand. Rehashing it, however, is overthinking.

- **Where is my focus?** Is it seeking a solution or centering on the problem? Exploring strategies to lose those last 10 pounds is problem-solving. Thinking about how awful you looked at the office party or imagining yourself featured in an exposé about morbid obesity is overthinking.

- **Are my thoughts accomplishing anything?** Are you finding viable solutions, or are you imagining their disastrous outcomes? If you are contemplating valid ways to fix the issue, you are problem-solving. If you are analyzing each result and getting stuck on ways each one *might* go wrong, you are overthinking.

In moments when you are seeking answers, if you find you are truly problem-solving, don't stop until you arrive at a solution that is doable, will achieve your goals, and can be put into action. If, however, you find you are actually overthinking, acknowledge that misstep and make the conscious choice to stop the process. You may need to revisit some of the strategies we've discussed in previous chapters to help you do that—and do it consistently—but once you achieve *this* solution to *this* problem, you'll be surprised at the renewed intellectual capacity you'll discover and the worthwhile activities you'll have the freedom to enjoy.

TO REITERATE: OVERTHINKING IS NOT PROBLEM-SOLVING

This misconception is such a problem, I feel we must revisit it. Back in Chapter 1, we established that, contrary to the popular defense of overthinking, it is *not* problem-solving. It is quite the opposite because, as you constantly overanalyze and rerun problems through your mind, you do arrive at solutions, but you don't stop there. You don't make a decision and take action. You think none of the options are good enough or that they might be good, but there must be something better. Perhaps perfectionism kicks in, and you refuse to accept any that will work because you are determined to find the absolute best way possible, without question.

As you can see, nothing gets accomplished when you overthink. When the analytical takes over, it easily identifies weak spots, goes down those rabbit holes, and creates new problems. Then, you start trying to solve those issues. It could potentially deprive you of several hours of productive activity. It could damage relationships by routing your focus to nonessential imaginings and keep you from tending to and nurturing those connections. It could result in missed opportunities, a lost job, confusion about what the real issue is, depression and guilt for trapping yourself in such futile intellectual waste, anxiety about the new problems you've launched, and many, many more negative effects on your mental, physical, and social states.

Remember the theoretical problem of forgetting to buy groceries for your weekend brunch with friends? How did the healthy problem-solver respond?

- They realized there was a problem.
- They brainstormed possible solutions.
- They stopped thinking about it when they came to one that would work.
- They put the solution to task, and they moved on from the problem.

Look at the third point: **They stopped thinking about it** when they came to one that would work. Problem-solving involves recognizing a solution and acknowledging its effectiveness. It requires you to let go of concerns that something else is just around the corner of your mind and the desire to keep chasing it. Does this solution resolve the issue? If yes, will it satisfy all requirements? If yes, will it produce any negative effects—any real, legitimately adverse effects? If not, what steps can be taken to implement it?

Continue to the fourth point: **They put the solution to task, and** they **moved on** from the problem. They committed to their decision and set it into action. At that point, they stopped thinking about it. They stopped ruminating over the past event that led to the problem. They stopped worrying about possible future outcomes that could result from this decision (that most likely won't happen). They changed gears and got off the merry-go-round, and when they did, they added no anxiety to their day and felt no depression or guilt. Instead, they felt confident and satisfied in their ability to reason and work out a practical application. And you can do this too!

FIVE STAGES OF PROBLEM-SOLVING

According to Al Pittampalli of the *Harvard Business Review*, there are five stages of solving problems (2019). He says all individuals proceed through these steps whenever they are faced with an issue that they must resolve on their own and that we usually do it without really thinking, hence why it's referred to as intuitive problem-solving. Now, if you're an overthinker, that may be hard to imagine, so let's walk through each stage one at a time to help you understand what it is your mind is experiencing:

- **Stage 1: Identify the issue.** The first thing you need to do is understand the problem. Define it. Note its parameters. Acknowledge its requirements. What question needs to be answered? Would you be able to communicate this problem to someone else? If not, then you may not fully understand it yourself, so keep exploring the issue until you're certain of what needs to be solved. As Steve Jobs wisely observed, by giving the problem a clear definition, you are well on your way to the solution (n.d.).

- **Stage 2: Think up solutions.** Consider known alternatives, but don't get too hung up on one.

Perhaps a standard fix could work, or maybe something similar that you've done before could apply, but think it all the way through. Each incident presents its own unique attributes, so you may need to be creative.

- **Stage 3: Assess possible solutions.** You've come up with some ideas. Now, it's time to evaluate them. Which one or ones best suit the situation? What are their strengths and weaknesses? Which will produce the most desirable potential outcome? Throw out any that definitely won't work. Continue to narrow down the options until you find what's right.

- **Stage 4: Make your choice.** After you've considered all the possibilities, you must decide which one you will pursue. Here's where overthinking can be a stumbling block because you may fall into distorted cognitions. You may worry about committing to any of them because they each have the potential to fail. You may be tempted to overanalyze, but remember that overthinking won't solve your problem. It will instead create more. So choose, but choose wisely.

- **Stage 5: Determine the steps to take to put the solution in action.** It's time to implement your decision. Again, you may be tempted to ruminate over past failures or worry about potential disappointments, but choose to move forward with your plan. What needs to be done to accomplish this solution? Does it require assistance or cooperation from anyone else? By what time or date does it need to be completed? What needs to be done now, and then next, and then after that until the desired result is achieved? Write it down and carry it out.

Pittampalli explains that we move through the stages unsystematically. For example, we might face the simple problem of choosing an ice cream flavor for dessert. That's pretty simple to define: What flavor do I want? You might skip over Stages 2 and 3, go directly to 4, and choose chocolate. But then you remember this store's chocolate wasn't chocolatey enough, so you bounce back up to Stage 2 to consider some alternatives. Yes, the strawberry here is definitely strawberry-y (Stage 3), so you ask the server to bring you some (Stage 4), and eat it (Stage 5)!

Though we slide back and forth between the phases as we come to a conclusive decision, we are not overthinking because we are determinedly seeking a solution, contemplating how to implement it, and putting an action plan in order.

PROBLEM-SOLVING STRATEGIES

To effectively and efficiently progress from defining a problem to implementing action steps, successful problem-solvers apply certain strategies and skills to get to the bottom of the issue. They observe, think, and analyze, but they do not overextend themselves in any of those areas.

An overthinker is probably aware that they overthink, and they likely want to stop, but it's not as simple as quitting cold turkey. Often, they feel helpless to get out of the loop they're stuck in. I know. I was an overthinker. Sandip Roy, medical doctor and founder of *The Happiness Blog*, which focuses on mental well-being, positive psychology, and, of course, happiness, explains that sheer willpower is not effective at breaking the cycle because it comes from the same areas of the brain that are stuck in the loop (2023).

Roy agrees with our assessment in Chapter 1 that the real problem is how to stop thinking and move on to action. He suggests the following strategies to put your thoughts to work:

- **As they say, practice makes perfect.** As you already know, habit-breaking doesn't happen overnight. Likewise, establishing new habits won't happen after doing just one mindfulness body scan, writing a single journal entry, or taking five deep breaths. You must practice them by doing them regularly if you want to see change. Roy recommends another technique to practice: As soon as you realize you've entered overthinking mode, intentionally distract yourself and consciously redirect your mind to a different thought or task.

- **The past is in the past; keep it there.** The past is unchangeable. You cannot go back in time and do things over again. Just thinking about it over and over is bad enough. Imagine reliving those memories over and over until you get it right. In truth, you are exhausting your mind and body with just the rumination as much as you would physically redoing the event. Allow yourself to move on. Mindfulness meditations are very helpful with this because when you're in a state of mindfulness, you work to accept the thoughts that come to mind without judging them or yourself for thinking them. This gives you the freedom to stop holding on to them and release them.

- **Solve a problem—a real one.** Set your mind on a problem at hand that needs an immediate solution. Try to choose a small problem, one that won't overwhelm you. You're trying to get away from angst-riddled worries, so look to something you can easily or quickly accomplish, like feeding the cat. Garfield's bowl is empty; it's dinner time. What will you do? You will dedicate your brain to finding the solution: Putting food in the bowl. Challenge yourself to shift your vision. Stop looking inward at the spinning gears and see something tangible you can do something about.

- **It may sound cliché, but it really is beneficial to have an attitude of gratitude.** There are two types of ruminations: intrusive, which occurs automatically as a result of a specific incident, and deliberate, which occurs as an intentional attempt to understand the purpose of a specific incident. Post-traumatic stress disorder (PTSD) results from intrusive rumination, but deliberate rumination can bring healing—referred to as post-traumatic growth (PTG)—after a traumatic event. PTG brings positive change in response to a life-changing crisis and manifests in gratitude and appreciation for life as those affected find new meaning. So practice feeling grateful and expressing that thankfulness for today as well as events that have brought you to who you are right now.

Obstacles to Problem-Solving

Even if you think you've got this problem-solving thing mastered, any number of obstacles can interfere with reaching the desired solution to the matter at hand, such as the following (Cherry, 2023):

- **Making assumptions:** This can be a real issue for overthinkers because they already have a tendency to think they know what other people are thinking and anticipate their response before a topic has even been broached. As an overthinker, you may also make assumptions about the solutions you're considering. If you don't stay focused on finding a resolution, you can easily slip into the loop of overanalysis by allowing the potential constraints and obstacles to prevent you from taking action on any option.

- **Fixating on standard answers:** In this case, you automatically default to the way you would normally see this problem handled, and you don't dare contemplate anything besides the customary solution. That might not work in this particular situation, though. Perhaps other factors are at play. Don't let this fixation prevent you from exploring different options or getting creative and thinking up your own ways to solve the problem. Put your adaptability skills to use.

- **Being misled by faulty information:** The problem you're presented with can become complicated when irrelevant information is thrown in. Whenever you are facing a challenge, be sure to distinguish between what is relevant to the issue and what can throw you off-topic. Discard data that misleads or unnecessarily makes the problem more complex than it really is.

- **Sticking with what you know:** Maybe you've faced a similar problem in the past, and you know of a solution that worked then, so you want to commit to that one right away. Pause! Remember what we said about this in Stage 2 of problem-solving? Just because it worked before doesn't mean it is right for this specific issue. Going with something you know may be convenient, but you need to fully assess the matter before jumping into anything. Always look for and be open to alternative ideas. You don't necessarily have to invent an entirely new concept every time, but innovation could be your best friend here. It could be that a previous option will work if it is tweaked a bit or customized to suit the situation.

How do you overcome these struggles without slipping back into your overthinking habits? How can you improve your problem-solving skills and strengthen your resolve?

SHARPEN YOUR PROBLEM-SOLVING SKILLS

A problem occurs when there is something we want out of life, but the way to achieve or acquire it is not clear. Problems can be large or small and about anything imaginable. We've talked about some big ones, like a country's economic struggles, and we've giggled at some small ones, like choosing an ice cream flavor. It doesn't matter what you're trying to figure out; you need to be able to progress through the process effectively. To do that, sometimes you'll need to pull from other skills you possess, and sometimes you might need to sharpen those tools.

You've already learned the stages of problem-solving: defining the problem, exploring and assessing possible solutions, choosing one, and then putting it into action. The most integral part of that procedure is to fully understand the problem. If you miss the point, you'll miss the target completely, and your solution will fail miserably.

The Importance of Asking Questions

Remember the Socratic method we mentioned in Chapter 3? By this method, instead of the teacher simply filling the student's mind with information, the student is encouraged to ask questions from their own curiosity to get as complete an understanding of the material as possible. Asking questions leads to finding answers you didn't know were there.

Leaders ask questions to make sure their subordinates are paying attention and enhance their own effectiveness. Followers ask questions to better grasp what they're being instructed to do or know. Whichever your position, asking questions will get you the clearest picture of the situation you're in and help you find solutions to problems.

Julia Brodsky of *Forbes* magazine suggests that when you ask questions, you are more likely to take ownership of your learning. You gain confidence in your abilities, have more courage to overcome fears created by overthinking, and assuredly demonstrate your comprehension (2020). This outcome is logical because you have, in effect, done your research and can present your solution with information to substantiate it. You haven't just come up with things you'd like to see happen based on your personal opinions or biases.

No person has all the answers, not even the greatest minds of all time. Even geniuses must ask questions. No one is born with all of life's knowledge. Somewhere in time, though, people became ashamed of what they didn't know, and it became an embarrassment to make inquiries. I hope this doesn't describe you! I hope, instead, that you feel empowered by gaining new insight and are excited to share what you learn.

The *Power of Positivity* promotes these 11 reasons why it's important to ask questions (Ethans, 2020):

- **It's how you learn.** I've said it before, and I stand by the statement. You don't know a lot. I don't know a lot! The only way to find that information is to query it, look into it, and go get it. You do this by asking questions.

- **It lets you turn things inward.** Sometimes, the answers are inside you, and you just need to reflect upon the issue. Maybe it's not new knowledge you're after but something you already possess that you need to bring to the surface.

- **It helps you understand the problem you're trying to solve.** Ding, ding, ding! This is what we're after in problem-solving. Remember that if you don't understand the issue, you won't be able to effectively resolve it.

- **It equips your brain.** You gain three important things when you ask questions: wisdom, flexibility, and positive thinking. Wisdom is procured knowledge you utilize maturely. Flexibility is being able to access stored information without resorting to faulty ways of thinking (like distorted cognitions and dysfunctional thoughts). Positive thinking leads to improved self-confidence, which is accompanied by renewed self-esteem and stronger self-compassion.

- **It provides more accurate solutions.** Because you're not solely relying on what you know or how you feel, you have research and resources to back up your propositions and give your solutions substance.

- **It prohibits judgment.** Instead of making biased assumptions or deeming something inadequate, you discover facts based on educational pursuit. It also slows you down and makes you more thorough.

- **It prevents pride.** Asking questions usually requires you to interact with someone else or at least to interact with research someone else has done. This keeps you from puffing yourself up as the only expert in the subject on the planet and keeps you humble.

- **It makes people like you.** Because it reveals a vulnerability—you don't know everything and you're not afraid to seek out what you don't know—you appear more relatable to others, and they will be more likely to interact with you in a comfortable manner.

- **It makes you a better-liked and more approachable leader.** Not only do you reveal a vulnerability, but you also express an interest in others when you ask questions of those who work for you. It makes your subordinates feel like you will listen to and care about what they have to say.

- **It can get you what you want from others.** That sounds a bit manipulative, but it's not intended that way. By posing your questions in the right way, you can be more direct and obtain more precise information.

- **It makes you ponder.** Sometimes you get an answer you weren't expecting, and it forces you to take a new look at the situation. You may gain a new perspective and discover solutions that would otherwise have never entered your mind.

Keep this Chinese proverb in mind as you seek the knowledge you're after: "The wise ask questions to become wiser. And the fool becomes wise by asking the right questions" (Victorscorner, 2016).

Sharpening Those Skills

The first skill to sharpen is your ability to interpret the issue. When presented with the problem, grab a pen and paper or open a word processor or note app on your device and write what you know. Don't rely on your memory to store your thoughts. Get them out in a tangible form that you can visually perceive and refer to them throughout the problem-solving process. This will also help you to not spin the wheels of your mind and get stuck overthinking any aspect.

After you've recorded what you already know about the topic, ask yourself and others who are knowledgeable about it for more details. Go beyond the basics, like timeframe, financial constraints, and other conditions, and get to the nitty-gritty.

Ask yourself questions. Why is this a problem? Who will the solution benefit? What is the desired outcome for those involved? Do we need a short-term fix or a permanent result? Who will be involved in completing the action steps? Write down and answer as many questions as you can think of before you even try to come up with solutions.

Ask others questions. Remember that you don't possess all knowledge. Sometimes, you need insight from others who have different expertise. Find out what they know about the issue and see if they can clarify things or give you something that will help you clarify the problem and understand what a proper solution might look like. The more thorough you are at the beginning, the more fluently you will flow through the rest of the process.

Once you fully understand the problem at hand, pick that pen back up (or return to your device) and brainstorm. Again, get it out of your head so you aren't tempted to ruminate or overanalyze. Simply put the possibilities down on paper.

Ask more questions. Once you have possible solutions, analyze them and rule out ineffective ones. Before long, you'll arrive at a solution you can be confident about because you have acquired sufficient background and foresight to move forward. Now, put the steps in order and charge ahead.

You may have noticed a theme here: *Ask questions!* When you master this ability, you will possess one of the sharpest tools in your problem-solving kit. There are, however, other ways to improve your deliberating proficiency.

As Albert Einstein once said, "You can never solve a problem on the level on which it was created" (n.d.). So let's take a step outside of traditional thinking and take a look at those options:

- **Adult Block Play:** This functional format brings fun into problem-solving. Initially designed for use in adult workshops to encourage teamwork, interaction, and discussion, it has also become a popular tool to build critical thinking skills in children ages six and up by encouraging imagination to complete each kit. Using 3D tangibles, it encourages you to think differently because it involves tactile touch and physical motion as well as intellectual reasoning.

- **Design sprint:** This is intended for team cooperation in corporate settings in which a design needs to be conceptualized, tested, and presented to customers in an accelerated time frame. However, it can be used by individuals who want to develop their problem-solving abilities too. To utilize this method, set an incontestable timeline, like five days for something complex or shorter if it's a simpler problem. Divide that into blocks of time and devote one problem-solving stage to each block. Challenge yourself to move through the stages quickly and arrive at your action steps without requiring an extension. This rapid sprint through the process will not allow you time to overthink or overanalyze.

- **Active listening:** Active listening is an important skill to possess in life in general. It strengthens relationships, improves job performance, and in regard to problem-solving, it provides clarity about the problem at hand. You can practice active listening anywhere and with anyone. You can even practice it while watching TV! Remove distractions, turn off your cell phone and other technical devices, and focus all attention on the person with whom you are interacting. Allow the other person to speak and fully express their message before you say anything. In fact, pause a moment before responding to make sure they are done speaking and give yourself time to absorb what they said. In your own words, repeat the idea they expressed to you and *ask questions* to enhance your understanding. You can take turns with a friend to work on your communication skills as well. If you have no one to partner with, turn on the television. Pay close attention to what a particular character is saying. Hit the pause button to stop the scene and pretend you are the one they were talking to. Then, apply the same advice as presented above. Rewind and play the scene again to see if you listened well enough to take in all the information.

- **Change your mindset:** Sometimes, we can become comfortable in our own ways of solving problems. However, as mentioned in an earlier section, that can impede the problem-solving process by keeping you locked into limited options. Allow yourself to be creative. *Ask yourself questions* that are outside the standard answers. Better yet, *ask other people* how they'd approach the issue or research the topic to discover how experts have handled similar topics. Remember that not all the answers are in your mind, and you may need to reach beyond your own understanding and potentially change the way you think about the issue in order to find an effective solution.

- **Mind mapping:** This technique helps you simplify your objective. You create a visual thought tree, writing your central topic—in our case, the problem—in the center of the page and branching off supporting ideas from that core focus. It is very simplistic. You use keywords instead of complete sentences or paragraphs to draw a plat of your problem-solving process. This is a great way to narrow down your options because you can physically cross out unfavorable ones or circle those with potential. Again, by combining physical motion with cerebral contemplation, your mind acts more decisively and presents more profitable results.

Store these tools in your problem-solving kit. Utilize them to help you break free from your overthinking habits and to build your self-confidence and productivity.

CHAPTER 6:

MINDFUL COMMUNICATION

We have two ears and one mouth so that we can listen twice as much as we speak. –Epictetus

In Chapter 2, we discussed mindfulness at length. Mindfulness is the mental state of being in the moment. It is an active practice, meaning you're not in a vacant mind frame, but you are intentionally releasing your inner angst without judgment and enhancing your awareness. It means awakening your mind to the present without regretting past actions and behaviors (ruminating) or anticipating future failures (worrying).

There are many methods of achieving those goals. None is more correct than any other, and though some techniques may be more effective for you, there is no singular right way to practice mindfulness. No matter which you choose, you will inevitably benefit from positive effects, like infrequent overthinking, less anxiety, reduced depression, lowered blood pressure, and improved cognition.

In this chapter, we are going to hone in on a particular element: mindful communication. This is a mindfulness practice, but it is also a concept you can carry into other areas of your life to improve interpersonal skills as well as *inner*personal treatment of yourself. It will help you develop relationships with others and acceptance of yourself as you learn to avoid criticism and cynicism. We'll also examine how enhancing awareness of the present moment keeps you from overthinking.

HOW DO YOU MINDFULLY COMMUNICATE?

Mindfulness trains your mind to act with intention while reducing the likelihood of reacting recklessly. While it greatly impacts your inner world, mindfulness also benefits your external interactions. Mindful communication increases understanding between you and the person you're socially involved with at the moment. Better comprehension eliminates misunderstandings and faulty judgments and leads you both to a more trusting relationship. Whether it is a personal involvement or a business associate, improved connections benefit all involved.

Jaquelyn Ikonomov of the American Institute for Stress tells us that to engage in a mindful conversation, we must be fully present in it (2021). We must apply the active listening skills we learned about in the previous chapter. First, disconnect from all electronic devices and remove yourself from distractions. Then, concentrate on what the speaker is saying without interjecting your own opinions. It is necessary to practice this technique so that when you encounter someone in a real-life situation, you are prepared to plug your attention into their message with all your effort.

To practice mindful listening, you may want to turn on soothing music or nature sounds. Allow yourself to focus on the musical pattern or the waves of the sea, surrender to them, and let them flow through your thoughts and carry away any negativity or faulty thinking that resides there. Keep your thoughts on the sounds and not on ruminations or worries. This is not the time to problem-solve or overthink.

Turning It Inward

Mindful communication impacts more than just intersocial dealings. When you turn it inward, you gain much mental improvement. As one expert describes, it "boosts our emotional immune system" and minimizes the impact of the ups and downs we experience (Chapman, 2019). Mindfulness teaches you to maintain an equilibrium of your feelings. You attain mental stability by practicing it regularly.

Here are some ways you can benefit from applying mindful communication to your own thoughts, reflections, and deliberations:

- **You create awareness of what thoughts are running through your mind.** This enables you to determine whether they are helpful or harmful, accurate or faulty. You can assess each one and boot to the curb those that lead to negative or errant ideas or that trigger overthinking.
- **You catch yourself entering a loop.** Because mindfulness enforces awareness of the present moment, you are able to recognize the moment you start to ruminate or worry. Instead of triggering the overthinking cycle, it will prompt you to practice your mindfulness techniques or other methods

you've learned throughout this book to put a stop to it before it consumes you.

- **You increase your awareness** of the cycle, the ruminations, the cognitive distortions, and the other negative effects that accompany overthinking. But because you have obtained effective techniques, such as mindfulness practices, you've learned to prevent them, stop the loop if it has already begun, and escape the mind trap.

RED LIGHT, YELLOW LIGHT, GREEN LIGHT

Susan Gillis Chapman of *Mindful* hosts workshops for participants who want to improve their mindful communication skills. She utilizes a simple metaphor to help them recognize whether they are in a closed, in-between, or open channel of communication: a traffic light. When communication has shut down, the light is red, when it's on the verge of shutting down, it's yellow, and when it's open, it's green. Chapman explains that when we close down our communication channels, we become defensive, shy away from others, and isolate ourselves (2019). But mindful communication helps us to be aware of which state we are in—or are entering—and helps us shift gears to avoid a wreck of emotions for both parties.

Red Light

Just like the traffic light, the red zone is a stopping place. Metaphorically, you have not only hit the brakes, but you've also shifted into park and turned off the car. If the light changes, it may take you a moment to get going again because you have put yourself in such a terminal state of communication. In the red light zone, you're likely to do the following:

- **Justify your defensiveness.** You hold onto your beliefs tightly. We all do. If someone infringes on your long-held opinions, you might feel that you are right and they are wrong, end of discussion. You'll convince yourself that the relationship wasn't important, keep your own interests first, and write off the connection.

- **Feel distrustful of others.** If someone violates your convictions, you may see their views as irreconcilably different from yours, possibly even threatening to your viewpoint. You will not feel secure in furthering the relationship because you will not trust their sentiment.

- **Become manipulative or controlling.** In this closed state, you may isolate yourself from others. This, of course, can lead to loneliness and desperation for human contact. But because you are feeling defensive and untrusting, you could attempt to hold the reins of the relationship until you determine it's safe to move forward.

- **Fear the isolation you've placed yourself in.** Regardless of how confident you are in the situation, the sense of isolation can be terrifying. Worries can rear their ugly head: *Can I really survive in this world with no one by my side? Who will come to my aid if I need help?*

- **Grow more rigid and out of touch.** Although you may become concerned about your isolation, you suppress those fears. You keep up a facade, but it only reinforces your reluctance to connect to others and makes you lose touch with your internal homeostasis. You may even begin to feel physical symptoms like strained muscles, headaches, or digestive issues as this state of being impacts your overall well-being.

Yellow Light

A yellow traffic light illuminates between red and green to indicate caution. Likewise, a metaphoric yellow in the communication channel is a warning zone. Chapman says this is the place we don't usually want to go: It's where "the ground falls out from beneath our feet, when we feel surprised, embarrassed, disappointed—on the verge of shutting down" (2019). When you are here, you might do the following:

- **Question why you're here.** You'll start to analyze your motivation and try to understand what caused you to close communications in the first place, and you start to wonder if it's worth your while to reopen them.

- **Experience sudden, unexpected transitions.** Just like the yellow traffic light can catch you off guard and seem to morph without warning, in this zone, you might abruptly lose trust in someone or in yourself and sense a startling cognizance of self-consciousness.

- **Give pause to the situation.** Just as it is more advisable to follow the traffic law and prepare to stop instead of speeding ahead into the red, it is crucial to learn to hold steady in the metaphoric yellow zone. Be curious, but practice mindful conversation as you prepare to reopen the communication channels.

Green Light

While the green traffic light signals you to proceed through the intersection, it is still advisable to do a quick check to make sure it's safe to do so. Look once more to the left, right, and across the lanes to make sure no one is running the light, that the way is clear, and that you can move ahead. Then, go into the green zone. When you go green, you may do the following:

- **Enter a state of knowing.** This is referred to as fluid awareness or fluid intelligence, and it means that you are letting go of your opinions and entering a new mind state. Simply put, in fluid intelligence, you think flexibly instead of holding on so tightly to your preconceived notions and beliefs.

- **Sense the flowing qualities of the world around you.** Your newfound fluidity allows you to explore your instincts, see if they were right or wrong, and test them out again.

- **Realize you don't have to remain in opposition.** You can have different viewpoints than another person without creating conflict. In this zone, you'll become aware that others' needs are simply different, not automatically wrong or dangerous. This will allow your mind to shift to a we-first state from your me-first state as you remember that humans are made to connect with others, and your personal survival depends on the well-being of your relationships.

- **Open communication back up.** Open communication returns you to the present moment. Even if the conflict is still there and the situation is awkward and uncomfortable, your willingness to share the joy and pain of others will restore the broken ties and advance you toward healing and growth.

STRATEGIES TO IMPROVE COMMUNICATION

It is common for communication between two people to break down. When it happens with a casual acquaintance, it's not such a big deal, but if it occurs between spouses, in intimate friendships, or within close working relationships, it can be devastating to both your mental well-being and your physical health.

Conflict is not always a bad thing. In healthy relationships, and when it is handled maturely and respectfully, it can lead to new understandings and fresh insights. However, sometimes the dispute can touch on sensitive areas and result in prolonged discord. If you remain in this strife, you may experience some of the following physiological effects:

- acne
- anxiety
- backache and reduced mobility
- depression
- eating disorders
- frequent illness and lowered immunity
- hair loss
- headaches or migraines
- heart attack or cardiac events
- sleeping disorders
- stomach ulcers or digestive tract complications
- tight, tense, sore muscles

When we are involved in a conflict, we tend to get headstrong and hold tightly to our position. But there are better ways to work through it, such as admitting when you're wrong, apologizing for your part in the dispute, and being empathetic instead of defensive. To resolve conflict—and, as an added benefit, improve your health—check out these additional strategies below to not only resolve existing conflicts but to prevent future ones from occurring:

- **Use "I" statements.** When you find yourself in a heated discussion, try to avoid directing your statements at your opponent with "you." They will receive your words as accusatory, like you're placing all responsibility for the argument and whatever led to it squarely on their shoulders. Instead, lead with "I" and express your feelings in response to what has occurred. As they say, it takes two to tango. It also takes two to clash.

- **Practice active listening.** Active listening requires you to physically hear the sounds being spoken and seek to understand what is being said. It is voluntary and takes effort on your part. It demands your focused attention. When discussing the conflict, remove distractions and turn off or silence your phone. Look your partner in the eye and maintain eye contact throughout the discussion. Pay attention to their body language and nonverbal cues and be aware of your own so as not to unwittingly incite an undesired reaction. Ask open-ended questions. Allow the other person time to finish saying their part, and do not interrupt. Pause to reflect before responding, and avoid passing judgment. Above all, be calm and compassionate.

- **Compromise.** Don't be determined to win the argument. Believe it or not, you might be in the wrong! Look for ways to work together to find solutions that meet everyone's needs. Usually, both participants want nothing more than to end the conflict, so compromise is more appealing than you might think. Neither should get what they want at the other's expense just to end the dispute. Find what benefits all involved, and both sides will be satisfied.

When I was still in the corporate world, I had worked tirelessly for months on a project that was crucial to the company's success. When it was finally completed, I expected to be praised for my hard work. Instead, my boss gave all the credit to my male colleague who had barely contributed.

I was so angry and hurt that I started to doubt my worth as an employee. It was hard to keep pushing myself when I didn't feel valued or supported by my employer. Though he wasn't aware of it, we were in conflict. I was still an overthinker at the time, so of course my mind started spinning. I was absolutely fuming, but at the same time, I was terrified to express myself. *I cannot believe he completely overlooked me! I did all the research. I assembled all the support. I put the report together. Jim did nothing! He was on vacation for two weeks while the project was in progress. He wasn't even here! Why does he get all the credit or any credit at all? Am I invisible here? I should really speak my mind. I should just go to the boss and tell him flat out that I did all that work. Me. Yes, a woman in the workplace did something of value. Oh, that will wake him up! Maybe I should go over his head to the supervisor and let him know his female employees are overlooked and undervalued. Maybe I should file a lawsuit. Maybe I should take my story to the news stations!*

The more fired up I got, the less I wanted to back down. I had no interest in having a calm conversation. I wanted my due recognition and fair treatment. I did not want to suggest any compromise. Compromise? What was there to compromise? I did the work, and I deserve to be acknowledged. I had no interest in listening to any excuse the boss would inevitably make either. As far as I was concerned, nothing he could say would be worth my effort to hear. I was ready to storm into his office with all the "I, I, I" statements cycling through my brain.

I feared the conflict, though. And that was probably a good thing because it likely saved my job.

Though I was still an overthinker, I was starting to investigate how to break that habit. I was taking a long time to approach my boss. I was indecisive about how to do it or if I should even take the risk. To prepare to face the conflict, I practiced the fear hierarchy on smaller matters (Cuncic, 2021):

- **I said "no" to a less significant matter.** When a friend asked to borrow my high-brand handbag, I declined.

- **I took a deep breath and complained about unsatisfactory service**. The meal I ordered at a restaurant was not the one I received, so I sent it back.

- **I created a new problem for myself.** I tried to pay for a purchase at a department store with an expired credit card that I knew wouldn't work.

- **I asked someone not to do something.** Someone at the library was playing music on a speaker instead of using headphones while I was trying to focus on my research, and I politely asked them to turn it off.

After processing this advice, and working through various real-life conflict scenarios, I decided to schedule a meeting with my boss to discuss my contributions to the project and how I felt about the situation. I presented him with evidence of my contributions and explained how it felt to be disregarded. He listened and apologized, and we worked together to establish clearer guidelines for recognizing employee contributions. After that, I felt more valued and supported in my role and empowered to diplomatically handle disputes.

WHY MINDFUL COMMUNICATION WORKS

Because mindful communication keeps your focus on what's immediately in front of you—that brief, fleeting moment we call the present—you are unable to look back or peek ahead. We sometimes take it for granted, but remaining in the now requires a lot of effort.

If you are hanging on every word that comes out of your partner's mouth right now, you cannot ruminate. If you want an effective conversation, you must hear with your ears and your mind. That means if your mind is back in the museum three days ago when you dropped your coffee and the splash came inches from ruining a 200-year-old painting, you can't take in the details of your partner's job promotion. If you're rehashing *I'm going to be banned from the museum! Because of me, they'll change all the rules about food and drinks. All future visitors will roll their eyes and talk trash about me even though they don't know me and don't know what happened and don't know that it didn't actually get on the painting but it almost did and...*, you won't know that they're proud of their achievement and excited about the opportunities it will bring. Because you haven't heard a word. When they bring the subject up again later and you stare blankly, they'll be hurt by your neglect and will interpret it as unconcern.

Maybe your mind would go forward instead of backward. You may be tempted to jump ahead of your partner. You might hear the keyword "promotion" and start thinking you can afford a new house with the pay raise they'll get. Your mind could just as easily take a time machine to the future as it did to the past, and you could end up worrying over *We've got to sell this house! It's such a mess. We have to declutter and make it ready to be shown by a Realtor. Oh, I've always wanted to move to that neighborhood on the lake. We'll finally be able to do it! What if the promotion doesn't go through? What if the raise isn't big enough? I wonder when it will take effect.* And you will end up damaging the relationship instead of building upon it.

However, if you have tuned in, your mind can't wander. If you're hearing all the joy your partner is sharing, and you're learning about the hard work they've put into their accomplishments, you will be proud of them and share their joy. You will automatically be interested because you *do care*, and you have remained attuned to the message they are sending. Their appreciation will expand, and both of you will feel a stronger connection.

Mindfulness gives you the ability to steady yourself when you have been hurt or are disappointed and prevents you from aggravating the issue. It brings about cooperation by encouraging healthy interactions.

CHAPTER 7:

OVERCOMING PERFECTIONISM

STOP OVERTHINKING

MIA PARKER

In a moment of decision, the best thing you can do is the right thing to do, the next best thing is the wrong thing, and the worst thing you can do is nothing. –Theodore Roosevelt

We touched on perfectionism as a cause of overthinking in Chapter 1, and I've been thinking about it ever since! All kidding aside, this is an issue that stops many people in their tracks, myself included.

I won't hesitate to admit that I'm a perfectionist. In many ways, it helps me; in others, it hinders. When it works for me, it prompts me to persist in my work and present my absolute best effort. This applies to relationships, hobbies, and even housework too. But perfectionism is dangerous because it's very easy to cross the line from wanting to do a good job to being obsessed that it could be better. If you're not careful, you'll find yourself unable to carry out a project to completion.

QUALITIES OF A PERFECTIONIST

Perfectionists can't seem to arrive at acceptable solutions because, in their minds, there's always a better answer. They drive themselves into preoccupation with the topic at hand thinking and rethinking, analyzing and overanalyzing, looking, searching, scanning, and raking through every detail trying to find perfection, flawlessness, primeness, ultimate impeccability… I can't find the right word for it! You see what I did there? That may seem a silly demonstration, but it's how perfectionism drives an individual to keep on going. I found several adequate words to communicate the message, but the pursuit of perfection kept me perusing the thesaurus.

What qualities define a perfectionist? Elizabeth Scott of *Verywell Mind* gives us some insight below (2023):

- **Being an all-or-nothing thinker:** Good enough is never sufficient for all-or-nothing thinkers. Like high achievers, perfectionists set lofty goals, but unlike high achievers, perfectionists never reach them. If the outcome is not a complete success, it's a complete failure. This way of thinking has no middle ground. While the high achiever can be satisfied with excellence, the perfectionist views excellence as mediocre. Anything less than perfect is flawed and can lead to worrying about its potential uselessness and ruminating afterward about the deficiencies in the conclusion.

- **Judging and criticizing yourself and others:** High achievers display a sense of pride in a job well done. They understand the work was hard, and they're proud of themselves for doing what it took to get it accomplished. They also encourage others and compliment their achievements too. However, perfectionists spot the mistakes every time. They see the imperfections in their own work and in that of others. A perfectionist has trouble seeing anything else and is highly critical of whoever's responsible for the perceived failure.

- **Being motivated by fear:** Most people have a healthy desire to achieve their goals and are content with the steps they take to move them toward those ends. Sometimes fear of missing a deadline or omitting pertinent information might give them a flutter, but overall, they get the job done and are satisfied. Perfectionists, however, fear anything less than perfection. If the deadline is met but some information was excluded, it's wrong. If the information is there, but it's insufficient to support the project, it's bad. If their work has any room for improvement, they keep trying to reach that prize.

- **Setting unrealistic standards:** Perfectionists tend to self-sabotage by setting their goals out of reach. They then suffer low self-esteem when they don't measure up because they feel that their actions are never good enough to meet the standards they themselves set.

- **Being upset about unmet goals:** Perfectionists don't accept failure easily. They tend to beat themselves up and enjoy a pity party of negative feelings when they fail to reach their high expectations. They struggle to move on, express less happiness, have higher levels of anxiety, and have lower levels of self-esteem than their counterparts because they are so dissatisfied with their inability to get everything just right. Striving for perfection is often related to high self-esteem, but perfectionists appraise themselves critically and end up in the dumps.

- **Fearing failure:** Perfectionists have a stronger fear of failure than those with a healthy sense of motivation. Because they put so much pressure on themselves to produce impeccable results, and because, to them, anything less than perfection is inadequate, failure is a menacing monster.

- **Putting things off:** The perfectionist's screeching inner critic combined with their formidable fear of failure equates to an inevitable propensity to procrastinate. Though avoidance of what needs to be done can delay or even prevent productivity, perfectionists can so easily become consumed with worry that they'll produce something imperfect that they become immobilized and incapable of doing anything at all. This, of course, leads to greater feelings of failure, more disappointment, increased depression and anxiety, and defunct self-esteem as the procrastination persists at perpetuating the paralyzing cycle.

Are you a high achiever, or are you really a perfectionist? Check all the boxes that apply:

You set unrealistic expectations for yourself.

You find fault in everything you do, even the small things.

You are quick to cast judgment over your thoughts, behaviors, and actions.

You fear failure.

You think good enough is not sufficient.

You dismiss compliments because you feel your work doesn't deserve notice—it could have been better.

You don't celebrate your success because your imperfect work didn't earn recognition.

You extend deadlines to give yourself more time to get it just right.

You hesitate to work with teammates because they might compromise the ideal.

You constantly compare yourself to others and judge yourself as inadequate.

You reject opportunities because you can't envision a perfect outcome and decide it's not worth the effort to give it a try.

Your negative self-talk shreds your efforts and convinces you the task is impossible.

You fail at relationships because they involve too many vulnerabilities and never work out as they're supposed to—aka, perfectly.

What's the score? Perfectionism 1, you 0?

Perfectionism is driven by internal pressures and incorrect assumptions that the rest of the world feels the same way you do. When you fall into this pattern, you succumb to the mind reading cognitive distortion in which you believe that you know what others think. Of course, it's a dysfunctional way of processing what goes through your mind. The catch-22 is that you continue to look to those same people for validation and approval. This keeps you caught in the web.

THREE TYPES OF PERFECTIONISM

Perfectionism exists in three domains: self-oriented, other-oriented, and socially prescribed. The common thread that binds them is perception. Each has to do with how you or others perceive the world around you and how you project those views onto others.

- **Self-oriented:** This type of perfectionism is wrapped up in the individual. You impose an unreasonable striving for perfection upon yourself. In doing so, you paralyze yourself and make it virtually impossible to achieve any level of success because you deem your efforts flawed.

- **Other-oriented:** Here, you extend the limitations you've placed on yourself to others. You expect everyone else to adhere to the same standards of perfection you require from yourself. In doing so, everyone fails you.

- **Socially prescribed:** With socially prescribed perfectionism, you perceive expectations of perfection from others. You believe it is expected of you from anyone you encounter, whether they be in real life or in the virtual world of social media.

Science has shown that over the last 30+ years, perfectionism has become a plague among young people. Socially prescribed perfectionism is the leading cause, and it is the driving force behind self- and other-oriented manifestations as well.

The authors of a 2019 study analyzed data from 41,641 college students across the United States of America, Canada, and the United Kingdom. They used the Multidimensional Perfectionism Scale, which measures 45 items on a 7-point scale to determine the participants' levels of perfection in each of the three dimensions discussed above. They discovered alarming statistics that revealed that between 1989 and 2016, occurrences of all three types increased: self-oriented by 10%, other-oriented by 16%, and socially prescribed by 33% (Bergland, 2018).

The authors of the study expressed great concern over their findings, especially over the potential mental and emotional harm perfectionism can impart. According to a 2017 World Health Organization report, young people in all three countries involved in the survey are experiencing dramatically higher numbers of anxiety disorders, depression, and suicide ideation than they were just a decade prior. They also report more loneliness, eating disorders, and body dysmorphia (preoccupation with an imagined physical defect).

The authors say more research is needed to confirm the correlation, but there is no doubt that increased social media usage is highly influential on the increased desire to be perfect. Educational performance and job competition are some other contributing factors to the rise in perfectionism among millennials. Thomas Curran, one of the study's authors, says that young people today are pressured by society to compete intensely with one another. Because of this, they feel perfectionism is the only means of achieving the highest status and top worth (Bergland, 2018).

OVERTHINKING AND ANALYSIS PARALYSIS

The Center for Advancing Health provides some startling statistics: 31% of college students have an anxiety diagnosis, 41.7% of adults ages 18–29 suffer from some form of anxiety, 27.3% of all American adults have anxiety problems, and 7.1% of the U.S. population has a social anxiety disorder (Julia, 2023). These numbers are significant indicators that either the chicken or the egg is overpopulating! Which is driving which—overthinking or anxiety—we don't quite know, but it's obvious they aggravate each other's condition.

An official diagnosis of an anxiety disorder confirms that the person struggling encounters much more serious symptoms and ill effects than simply getting nervous or feeling jittery when faced with an uncomfortable situation. These symptoms don't just go away. They can grow worse over time, their triggers can change, and the person's physical health can be affected by long-term detriment. The sufferer often requires therapeutic treatment and medication to properly manage the disorder, and depending on the severity of the ailment, those treatments can potentially be a lifetime requirement.

Perfectionism results from trying to live up to your ideal internal image. As we've discovered, it can be motivated by a fear of failure, concern over how others perceive you, or an unsatisfiable longing to do or present the absolute best. Whether it's self-driven, other-driven, or socially prescribed, for a person with an anxiety disorder, the perceived shortcomings may distress both the mind and the body and leave them sick on multiple levels. They may become so distraught that they are unable to commit to decisions. As a result, their blood pressure rises, their heart palpitates, and their motivation plummets to nil.

Jodi Clarke of *Verywell Mind* labels this condition analysis paralysis (2022). I like that term! It's pretty accurate. It occurs when you move beyond thought and become overwhelmed. Here's something that overwhelmed me: The average person makes 35,000 decisions a day. If you're a perfectionist who is also an overthinker, I can easily see how you could become paralyzed by analyzing 35,000 choices.

When I was an overthinker—and a self-professed perfectionist, remember—one particular decision overwhelmed me into this condition. I had acquired the corner office of the finance division of a major corporation, and I had a lot of responsibility on my shoulders. In this position, I conceived a concept for accelerating our corporate growth both fiscally and as a global influence. I knew this would mean big changes in our division and some restructuring in other areas, but I was confident it would propel our group to international recognition and carry with it significant opportunities. I don't know how many decisions went into 1) defining the problem, 2) generating possible solutions, 3) assessing the solutions, 4) choosing an option, and 5) putting the action plan in order and carrying it out, but it felt like at least 35,000 were required for each step in the process.

As I said, I was still an overthinker at the time, so I went over each of those 35,000 decisions (times 5) what seemed like 35,000 times each. Yes, coworkers were involved, but as a perfectionist, I couldn't allow myself to fully rely on their input, and I had to evaluate and re-evaluate their input as well. *They might have missed something. They might have included the wrong information. They might have misapplied data. They might totally mess up my plan! I'll just go over it one more time. Then once more in case I missed something. What if I misapplied the data? What if I mess up my own plan?* Over and over and over it all went in my mind. I tossed and turned all night every night, analyzing, reworking, and searching for the ideal way to play this out. I had long passed good enough; I was hunting undeniable excellence, and it remained just out of my reach.

Then, one afternoon, right there in my cozy corner office, my head suddenly felt like it was lifting off my shoulders. At the same time, my vision telescoped, and the world around me shriveled into a distant, tunneled scene just beyond my fingertips. My heart pounded in my ears, and my breath left my chest.

The next thing I knew, EMTs were huddled around me, oxygen was forcing its way into my lungs, and machines were beeping and buzzing. Everything was surreal. I was physically present, but my mind was still cycling fast. *No! They can't take me to the hospital. Who will complete the project? Who will present it to the board? Who will carry it out? Who will make sure it's perfect?* And off I went a second time to the only place my mind could rest, unconsciousness.

It was a panic attack. My vitals checked out clear, but my mental state did not. I had succumbed to analysis paralysis, and if I didn't choose to make some major changes in my life right then and there, I might have succumbed to even more serious and potentially life-threatening maladies.

My breakdown likely saved my life. I had no intention of changing my trajectory. I had no intention of handing off my duties to anyone else. I had no intention of backing down, walking away, or doing anything to help myself until my mind made the decision for itself to pull the plug on perfectionism and grind the crazy train of self-destruction to a jarring halt.

Thus dawned a new beginning for me. I left the corporate world, sought new understanding, and discovered the me that had become buried by bad habits and misplaced priorities.

I don't ever want to experience that again, and I don't want you to go through it at all. Don't let analysis paralysis stifle you and leave you submerged in the mire of misery.

STRATEGIES TO OVERCOME PERFECTIONISM

Being a perfectionist is frustrating. No one is perfect, and no one can be perfect. No one makes perfect choices, and no one makes zero mistakes. It's challenging, and it's an exhausting mentality to maintain because perfection is always just out of reach. Even though your personal best may be miles ahead of your competitors, inside, you're not content with "best" because, to you, there's always room for better. And better. And better. Because of this relentless pursuit of faultless superiority, perfectionists end up achieving less and stressing more than high achievers who know when to determine a job has been completed to "well-done" satisfaction. See the proof for yourself in my story in the last section. I didn't achieve that goal of promoting our company to global notice. As a perfectionist, I left my position not empty-handed, but empty of that final task I intended to see through to perfect completion.

I had a major case of unhealthy perfectionism, and it nearly destroyed me inside and out. I had an excessive focus on control. I didn't even trust the input from my team. I was preoccupied with making every aspect inerrant, and it led to a complete loss of all control of my own mind as well as of my goals and even of the situations and people I managed. While that particular event isn't what brought my marriage to its conclusion, my perfectionism and persistent overthinking certainly took a major toll on the relationship, and it severely impacted my working affiliations as well.

Unhealthy perfectionism can not only make it difficult to achieve your goals; it can also destroy them.

If you notice perfectionist traits in yourself, don't despair. Don't worry, don't ruminate, and don't overthink! Recognizing the need for change is your first step. Understanding the possible negative effects of these tendencies can prod you toward a healthier approach to achieving your goals with less stress and more positivity.

The following strategies can help you arrive at that place:

- **Assess the value of your perfectionist traits.** You may think you need them, and you might be reluctant to give them up. Some may truly be beneficial because they may keep you producing to the best of your ability, but make sure they don't push you beyond the ability to commit to adequate solutions.

- **Write down your perfectionist tendencies.** If you can't do it in real time as the thoughts occur to you, jot them down in your journal each evening before you go to bed. This will help you be aware of what you're doing. By keeping them on paper in front of you, you will know to monitor those propensities and keep them in check.

- **Don't compare yourself to others.** If you already struggle with comparing yourself to yourself, you're sure to set yourself up for frustration, doubt, and negative self-talk by bringing others into the picture too.

- **Practice mindfulness.** We'll talk more about this below, but you can also refer to prior chapters of this book to refresh your memory of the many options available. The key is to devote a time and space to clear away distractions and focus on the present without worrying about the future or ruminating over the past.

- **Challenge negative thoughts.** Perfectionists tend to focus on the negative. They see what's wrong about a situation and how it can be improved rather than picking up on what's good and what works. Stop and look at your current circumstance.

What was done well—specifically, what did *you* do well? Make a conscious effort to notice and acknowledge successes and achievements both that you have done yourself and that those around you have accomplished too.

- **Fix your self-talk.** Be nice to *you*! As I said earlier, perfectionists spot the negatives. They're quick to insult themselves internally too. Wrestle that inner critic and put a muzzle on it. You are good. You are skilled. You are talented. You are successful. Don't let negative self-talk perpetuate unhealthy habits or destroy your self-esteem.

- **Take baby steps.** Don't overwhelm yourself by thinking you must fix everything all at once. This is too big of a task and will discourage you from reaching your goals. Instead, take baby steps. Write down your goals and determine the first part of the process. Focus only on the first thing! You will find that by tackling one small part at a time, you will gain confidence by seeing progress, and you will be inspired to continue.

- **Give up control over something small.** This will force you to let go of your perfectionist tendency to keep searching for what's better because you must stop and release your control over a situation.

- **Allow yourself to be flexible.** This may take some time. You've gotten yourself into a pretty established habit, and it might not be easy to release. By giving yourself permission to be imperfect, you will unload a very heavy burden and free yourself from the confines of compulsion.

Adopting a Growth Mindset

Developing a growth mindset is a sure way to help you drop the need for perfection and learn to embrace the you that you really are. According to Tchiki Davis of *Psychology Today*, "It is the belief that your basic abilities can be developed and improved through dedication and hard work" (2019). Davis tells us that by letting go of the comparison mindset we maintain as perfectionists, we can achieve at a high level without needing to meet the impossibly perfect ideal. If you have a growth mindset, you can enjoy problem-solving, challenges, and even partnering with others because you will not be fixated on realizing an unreachable goal: perfection. This usually occurs because you learn to value growth more than what others think or how they're performing. Because a growth mindset is about doing new things, you might not even know what the perfect ideal is for the opportunity at hand, and this frees you to explore, create, and discover more joy in everyday occasions.

Davis recommends the following ways to flip your fixed mindset over to one of growth:

- **Embrace imperfection in yourself and others.** Acknowledge that everyone has flaws, and you are no exception. Your imperfections make you unique.

- **Be brave.** Perfectionism is often driven by the fear of failure, but you can cast that aside and instead get excited about the new and unknown opportunities that lie ahead.

- **Be authentic.** Don't put up a facade of perfection. Those who know you know you're not really perfect, and guess what? They love you for it! Coworkers, friends, and other acquaintances appreciate genuineness. When you let your real self show, others will feel you are more approachable and relatable.

- **Stop scoring people by your perfection scale.** Someone's best effort may be their perfect. That doesn't make them less than, and your judgment of them definitely doesn't make you more than.

- **Remember that practice makes perfect.** In this case, we're not talking about the perfectionist's ideal. It means that you must put these techniques into practice in order to arrive at the desired goal: a growth mindset.

Mindfulness

Mindfulness practices are some of the most effective ways to beat perfectionism, to allow yourself to drop out of the obsession for optimum performance and be satisfied with—even proud of—your achievements.

Cheryl Jones of *Mindful* recommends the following 15-minute meditation to help you accept you for the you that you are (2021):

1. First, find your posture. Sit upright in a chair and close your eyes. Make sure your feet are flat on the ground. Let your arms hang loosely at your sides or rest your hands on your thighs. Gently pull your shoulder blades toward each other and keep your chin parallel to the floor. Feel the crown of your head lift toward the sky, relax your belly, and unclench your jaw.

2. Take a moment to notice what it feels like to stop and be in this purposeful posture. As you engage your intentions, appreciate your willingness to care for yourself and help yourself in this way.

3. Notice your breathing, but don't control or manipulate it in any way. Just breathe, right here, right now. Flow in and out with each breath.

4. Notice the breathing sensations and observe how the air moves in and out of your nose. Feel the air pass over your upper lip and the rise and fall

of your chest and ribs. Rest your attention on the sensations.

5. Don't block thoughts that pass through your mind. Allow them to proceed one by one, but don't judge them or label them good or bad, positive or negative, or helpful or harmful. Just observe them.

6. Shift your attention to what you're feeling in this moment. Don't assess your feelings. None are good or bad. All are acceptable and allowed to be in this moment.

7. Next, notice sensations within your body. Are you warm? Cool? Do you feel tingling or tightness? Can you feel your pulse? Are you hungry? Full? Be patient and kind to yourself. Don't be critical of any sensation but explore them with curiosity.

8. Reset your posture if it has shifted but stay attuned to your body as it is right now at this time and in this space.

9. Focus only on your breath now as we near the end of this practice. Continue three cycles of breathing, being as present as possible as you follow each inhale and exhale.

10. Softly flutter your eyes open and re-engage with your surroundings as you prepare to re-enter the day ready to bring awareness to all that you do.

Our brains are not designed to be fully mindful. The present moment is always ephemeral. As soon as you acknowledge its presence, it becomes the past. Our minds must be able to flow across time zones, so to speak, to keep us balanced between what has already happened and what we have to look forward to. This is why mindfulness is a *practice*, something we must intentionally determine to do to give our brains a break.

Imperfection is the norm. Relentlessly pursuing perfection is a fruitless endeavor. Improve your moment-to-moment well-being and allow yourself to be perfectly imperfect.

CONCLUSION:

FINDING HAPPINESS

The happiness of your life depends upon the quality of your thoughts. –Marcus Aurelius

I mentioned at the beginning of this book that along my journey, I found that I was not alone in the frustrating and debilitating habit of overthinking. I discovered many women on this path who were challenged by my same struggles, and my heart went out to them.

I found recovery. And believe me, if I can do it, you can too! So I made it my goal to help those women—and you—do the same. To achieve this end, I put my experiences to work as we considered the following:

- that overthinking means running the same thoughts through your head on repeat and that, despite popular defense, it is *not* problem-solving
- that overthinking is a terrible habit with potentially devastating effects on both your emotional and physical well-being
- that certain triggers cause you to overthink—to ruminate on past occurrences or worry about future possibilities—that you need to identify those triggers, and that you can put multiple techniques into action in order to *Stop Overthinking*

YOU DIDN'T OVERTHINK EACH CHAPTER AS YOU READ IT, DID YOU?

I sure hope you didn't overthink your way through this book, but it's quite possible that you did. I titled this subsection with a little humor because I know that breaking habits takes time. Unfortunately, crushing the overthinking cycle is not an overnight process. However, by regularly applying the strategies covered in this book, you will begin to notice changes in your thoughts and behaviors in a short amount of time.

In the first chapter, you learned that overthinking is a bit of a chicken-or-egg quandary: Experts cannot determine if overthinking came first and spawned anxiety, depression, and other emotional and mental disorders or if those ailments came first and resulted in the symptom of overthinking. Either way, ruminating and worrying do the mind and body absolutely no good.

A lot of the things you overthink can't be changed because they've already happened or you have no manner to affect change (like solving the world's problems, remember?). Some, though doable, are ineffectual because you won't let them out of your head. Instead of taking action, you continue to analyze the situation and search for better solutions.

It's important to remember how to get out of the loop you're stuck in! Remember to squish the ANTs, distract and redirect, see the big picture, be nice to yourself, and don't be afraid to ask for help.

Throughout the remaining chapters, we took a very detailed look at various techniques, strategies, and practices you can apply to your life to overcome the bad habit of overthinking.

A New Hope

My new hope for you is that you have found in this book a new understanding of what overthinking is, a new confidence that you can overcome it, and new ways to guide you through the process of breaking the overthinking habit and restoring your emotional well-being.

Is that your hope too?

I know you long for peace of mind. Overthinking is like an internal rebellion. Your mind interprets your decisions as the enemy and your rumination as the resistance. As they battle, they keep spinning your gears in overanalysis and repetition. You want off the wild ride of emotion and frustration with both feet planted solidly on "normalcy" (remember that term?) and productivity. As we progressed through each chapter, you read about several ways to bring this hope to fruition.

Some of the helpful solutions we discovered to help you do that included the following:

- Understanding the habit you're trying to break. You have gained new knowledge of the negative pattern of thinking that has disrupted your life, and you are now ready to defeat it.

- You learned several mindfulness practices that can help you calm your mind and body, redirect your thoughts, and put your body in motion by focusing on the moment instead of past ruminations and future worries.
- You learned how to recognize the distorted cognitions and dysfunctional thoughts that are keeping you stuck in the overthinking loop, and you found out about effective activities to restructure or reframe them.
- You learned that building resilience will help you bounce back from past events that you are tempted to ruminate about, and that by improving your self-esteem, you will increase your self-confidence, which will boost your self-compassion and enable you to help yourself out of this vicious cycle.
- You learned that overthinking is most definitely not problem-solving but is instead problem-causing. By considering and reconsidering your options or plans, you create new problems that didn't exist before. These waste your time and energy because they are futile and unnecessary. You learned proper problem-solving techniques to not only halt overthinking but also to arrive at firm decisions and stick to them.

- You learned to take those mindfulness techniques you discovered in Chapter 2 and apply them to communication. By doing so, you will improve communication with active listening and assertiveness to reduce overthinking and improve relationships.

- Finally, you learned to overcome a little problem that is a habit of its own but that also keeps your overthinking wheels spinning: perfectionism. Setting small, realistic goals, embracing imperfection, and adopting a growth mindset will help you be satisfied with your decisions and actions and keep you from constantly trying to make everything "better."

I am so happy that you have joined me on this journey! I sincerely hope you will put what you've learned into practice because I want you to rediscover *you* and to understand that you're not lost and you're not alone and you're not in a hopeless condition. I've introduced proven methods to help you escape the overthinking mind trap. I am living proof that they work!

At the end of the References list, I've included some helpful resources you can explore on your own as you take on this quest. If you have found this book beneficial, I'd love to hear your story and how it helped you, so please consider leaving your review on Amazon.

REFERENCES

About Jon Kabat-Zinn, an inclusive vision. (n.d.). Jon Kabat-Zinn. https://jonkabat-zinn.com/about/

Ackerman, C. (n.d.). *Automatic thought record.* Positive Psychology. https://positive.b-cdn.net/wp-content/uploads/Automatic-Thought-Record.pdf

Ackerman, C. (2017, September 29). *Cognitive distortions: 22 examples & worksheets (pdf).* Positive Psychology. https://positivepsychology.com/cognitive-distortions/

Ackerman, C. (2018, February 12). *Cognitive restructuring techniques for reframing thoughts.* Positive Psychology. https://positivepsychology.com/cbt-cognitive-restructuring-cognitive-distortions/

Arford, K. (2020, October 20). *10 science-based benefits of having a dog.* American Kennel Club (AKC). https://www.akc.org/expert-advice/lifestyle/10-science-based-benefits-dog/

Aristotle. (n.d.). *Hope quotes.* Brainy Quotes. https://www.brainyquote.com/quotes/aristotle_133079?src=t_hope

Bergland, C. (2018, January 3). Is the perfectionism plague taking a psychological toll? *Psychology Today.* https://www.psychologytoday.com/us/blog/the-athletes-way/201801/is-the-perfectionism-plague-taking-psychological-toll

Bergland, C. (2020, February 18). Self-compassion and meditation can yield better mental health. *Psychology Today.* https://www.psychologytoday.com/us/blog/the-athletes-way/202002/self-compassion-and-meditation-can-yield-better-mental-health

Bertin, M. (2015, October 6). *Mindfulness: The antidote for perfectionism.* Mindful. https://www.mindful.org/mindfulness-the-antidote-for-perfectionism/

Boyles, A. (2012, June 25). 20 uses for self-compassion. *Psychology Today.* https://www.psychologytoday.com/us/blog/in-practice/201206/20-uses-self-compassion

Brodsky, J. (2020, December 29). Why questioning is the ultimate learning skill. *Forbes.* https://www.forbes.com/sites/juliabrodsky/2021/12/29/why-questioning-is-the-ultimate-learning-skill/?sh=351ecdce399f

Brown, B. (2010). *The gifts of imperfection*. Hazelden Publishing. https://www.amazon.com/Gifts-Imperfection-10th-Anniversary-Features/dp/B085LLCPT5/ref=sr_1_1?crid=2YS6DXX24C765&keywords=The+Gifts+of+Imperfection&qid=1681591034&sprefix=%2Caps%2C360&sr=8-1&tag=aurum0a-20

Burton, N. (2015, October 19). Self-confidence versus self-esteem. *Psychology Today*. https://www.psychologytoday.com/us/blog/hide-and-seek/201510/self-confidence-versus-self-esteem

Chapman, S. (2019, July 4). *How mindful communication makes us more compassionate*. Mindful. https://www.mindful.org/stop-go-wait/

Cherry, K. (2022a, August 10). *What is cognitive behavioral therapy (CBT)?* Verywell Mind. https://www.verywellmind.com/what-is-cognitive-behavior-therapy-2795747

Cherry, K. (2022b, August 20). *What is homeostasis?* Verywell Mind. https://www.verywellmind.com/what-is-homeostasis-2795237

Cherry, K. (2022c, November 11). *Fluid vs. crystallized intelligence*. Verywell Mind. https://www.verywellmind.com/fluid-intelligence-vs-crystallized-intelligence-2795004

Cherry, K. (2022d, December 1). *The 6 types of basic emotions and their effect on human behavior*. Verywell Mind. https://www.verywellmind.com/an-overview-of-the-types-of-emotions-4163976

Cherry, K. (2023, January 3). *Problem-solving strategies and obstacles*. Verywell Mind. https://www.verywellmind.com/problem-solving-2795008

Clark, D. (2020, January 18). Are you an overthinker? *Psychology Today*. https://www.psychologytoday.com/us/blog/the-runaway-mind/202001/are-you-overthinker

Clarke, J. (2022, April 22). *What is analysis paralysis?* Verywell Mind. https://www.verywellmind.com/what-is-analysis-paralysis-5223790

Cohut, M. (2018, August 26). Dogs: Our best friends in sickness and in health. *Medical News Today*. https://www.medicalnewstoday.com/articles/322868

Cuncic, A. (2020, July 1). *Understanding cognitive restructuring*. Verywell Mind. https://www.verywellmind.com/what-is-cognitive-restructuring-3024490

Cunci, A. (2021, July 2). *How to overcome the fear of conflict with therapy.* Verywell Mind. https://www.verywellmind.com/how-do-i-get-over-my-fear-of-conflict-with-others-3024828

Currin, T., & Hill, A. (2019). Perfectionism is increasing over time: A meta-analysis of birth cohort differences from 1989 to 2016. *Psychological bulletin, 145*(4), 410–429. https://doi.org/10.1037/bul0000138

Davis, T. (2021, January 13). 6 science-based self-compassion exercises. *Psychology Today.* https://www.psychologytoday.com/us/blog/click-here-happiness/202101/6-science-based-self-compassion-exercises

Davenport, B. (2022, January 28). *Become a more mindful communicator with these 13 strategies and examples.* Mindful Zen. https://mindfulzen.co/mindful-communicator/

Donovan, L. (2016, September 21). *5 ways dogs help humans be healthier and happier.* American Kennel Club (AKC). https://www.akc.org/expert-advice/lifestyle/5-ways-dogs-help-humans-be-healthier-and-happier/

Dostoevsky, F. (1864). *Overthinking quotes.* Goodreads. https://www.goodreads.com/quotes/tag/overthinking

Einstein, A. (n.d.). *Albert Einstein quotes.* Brainy Quotes. https://www.brainyquote.com/quotes/albert_einstein_143191

Elmer, J. (2023, March 13). 5 ways to stop spiraling negative thoughts from taking control. *Healthline.* https://www.healthline.com/health/mental-health/stop-automatic-negative-thoughts#2-recognize-automatic-negative-thinking

Epictetus. (n.d.). *Communication quotes.* AZ Quotes. https://www.azquotes.com/quote/90291?ref=communication

Ethans, L. (2020, October 16). *11 reasons why it's important to ask questions.* Power of Positivity. https://www.powerofpositivity.com/ask-questions-why-important/

Ferguson, S. (2022, November 8). *Why self-esteem matters and tips to build yours up.* Verywell Mind. https://www.healthline.com/health/mental-health/high-self-esteem

Garrett, L. (2022, August 23). *What science says about the power of outbreath.* Mindful. https://www.mindful.org/what-science-says-about-the-power-of-the-outbreath/

Getting started with mindfulness. (2023, January 6). Mindful. https://www.mindful.org/meditation/mindfulness-getting-started/

Graham, L. (2014, August 20). How self-compassion beats rumination. *Greater Good Magazine.* https://greatergood.berkeley.edu/article/item/how_self_compassion_beats_rumination

Greater Good Science Center. (2010, April 14). *Jon Kabat-Zinn: What is mindfulness?* [Video]. YouTube. https://youtu.be/xoLQ3qkh0w0

Greenburg, M. (2019, March 31). Self-compassion may foster more secure attachment. *Psychology Today.* https://www.psychologytoday.com/us/blog/the-mindful-self-express/201903/self-compassion-may-foster-more-secure-attachment

Guided meditations. (n.d.). UCLA Health. https://www.uclahealth.org/programs/marc/free-guided-meditations/guided-meditations

Guy-Evans, O. (2023, March 6). *Primary and secondary emotions.* Simply Psychology. https://simplypsychology.org/primary-and-secondary-emotions.html

Hall, D. (2017, March 31). Mindful listening. *Psychology Today.* https://www.psychologytoday.com/us/blog/conscious-communication/201703/mindful-listening

Hartney, E. (2022, November 15). *10 cognitive distortions that can cause negative thinking.* Verywell Mind. https://www.verywellmind.com/ten-cognitive-distortions-identified-in-cbt-22412

Hewett, P., & Flett, G. (n.d.). *Multidimensional perfectionism scale and scoring.* https://hewittlab.sites.olt.ubc.ca/files/2014/11/MPS-RESEARCH-ONLY.pdf

Hoshaw, C. (2022, March 29). What is mindfulness? A simple practice for greater wellbeing. *Healthline.* https://www.healthline.com/health/mind-body/what-is-mindfulness

Howley, E., & Miller, A. (2023, January 19). How to stop overthinking and reduce anxiety. *U.S. News and World Report.* https://health.usnews.

com/wellness/mind/articles/proven-strategies-to-stop-overthinking-and-ease-anxiety-now

Ikonomov, J. (2021, February 10). *12 fun mindfulness exercises*. The American Institute of Stress. https://www.stress.org/12-fun-mindfulness-exercises

Jobs, S. (n.d.). *Steve Jobs quotes*. AZ Quotes. https://www.azquotes.com/quote/1059253

Jones, C. (2021, May 26). *A 15-minute meditation for self-acceptance*. Mindful. https://www.mindful.org/a-15-minute-meditation-for-self-acceptance/

Julia, N. (2023, January 5). *Anxiety statistics & facts: How many people have anxiety?* The Center for Advancing Health. https://cfah.org/anxiety-statistics/

Kane, R. (2022a, September 6). *33 mindfulness exercises for present-moment living*. Mindfulness Box. https://mindfulnessbox.com/mindfulness-exercises/

Kane, R. (2022b, December 8). *Printable mindfulness journal template (Get started fast)*. Mindfulness Box. https://mindfulnessbox.com/mindfulness-journal-template/

Kane, R. (2022c, December 8). *59 mindfulness journal prompts (printable)*. Mindfulness Box. https://mindfulnessbox.com/mindfulness-journal-prompts/

Kelly, O. (2020, August 14). *Obsessive compulsive disorder (OCD) and perfectionism*. Verywell Mind. https://www.verywellmind.com/ocd-and-perfectionism-2510483

Kristenson, S. (2021, October 2). *11 steps to develop the mindful communication practice*. Happier Human. https://www.happierhuman.com/mindful-communication/

Lamothe, C. (2023, February 15). 14 ways to stop overthinking. *Healthline*. https://www.healthline.com/health/how-to-stop-overthinking

Macdonald, C. (n.d.). *Monika Ardelt's model of wisdom*. The Wisdom Page. http://www.wisdompage.com/Ardelt01.html

MARC mindful meditations. (n.d.). UCLA Health. https://www.uclahealth. org/programs/marc/free-guided-meditations/guided-meditations

Marcus Aurelius quote. (180). Meditations, via Goodreads. https://www. goodreads.com/author/show/17212.Marcus_Aurelius

Mayo Clinic Staff. (2022a, July 6). *Self-esteem: Take steps to feel better about yourself.* Mayo Clinic. https://www.mayoclinic.org/healthy-lifestyle/ adult-health/in-depth/self-esteem/art-20045374

Mayo Clinic Staff. (2022b, July 14). *Resilience: Build skills to endure hardship.* Mayo Clinic. https://www.mayoclinic.org/tests-procedures/resilience-training/in-depth/resilience/art-20046311

Mayo Clinic Staff. (2022c, October 11). *Mindfulness exercises.* Mayo Clinic. https://www.mayoclinic.org/healthy-lifestyle/consumer-health/in-depth/mindfulness-exercises/art-20046356

Meraji, S., & Douglis, S. (2022, January 3). Stressed? Instead of distracting yourself, try paying closer attention. *National Public Radio (NPR).* https://www.npr.org/2021/12/21/1066585316/mindfulness-meditation-with-john-kabat-zinn

Merriam-Webster. (n.d.-a). *Compassion.* Merriam-Webster.com. Retrieved April 8, 2023, from https://www.merriam-webster.com/dictionary/ compassion

Merriam-Webster. (n.d.-b). *Equilibrium.* Merriam-Webster.com. Retrieved April 11, 2023, from https://www.merriam-webster.com/dictionary/ equilibrium

Merriam-Webster. (n.d.-c). *Homeostasis.* Merriam-Webster.com. Retrieved April 11, 2023, from https://www.merriam-webster.com/dictionary/ homeostasis

Merriam-Webster. (n.d.-d). *Overthink.* Merriam-Webster.com. Retrieved March 30, 2023, from https://www.merriam-webster.com/dictionary/ overthink

Merriam-Webster. (n.d.-e). *Overthinker (Alyssa Meier quote).* Merriam-Webster. com. Retrieved March 30, 2023, from https://www.merriam-webster. com/dictionary/overthink

Merriam-Webster. (n.d.-f). *Resilience.* Merriam-Webster.com. Retrieved April 8, 2023, from https://www.merriam-webster.com/dictionary/resilience

Merkur, D. (2023, February 16). *Meditation.* Encyclopedia Britannica. https://www.britannica.com/topic/meditation-mental-exercise

Mindful Staff. (2022, August 31). *The science of mindfulness.* Mindful. https://www.mindful.org/the-science-of-mindfulness/

Mindful Staff. (2023, January 6). *Getting started with mindfulness.* Mindful. https://www.mindful.org/meditation/mindfulness-getting-started/

Montgomery, J. (2012, September 30). Emotions, survival, and disconnection. *Psychology Today.* https://www.psychologytoday.com/us/blog/the-embodied-mind/201209/emotions-survival-and-disconnection

Morin, A. (2019, October 15). The difference between helpful problem solving and harmful overthinking. *Forbes.* https://www.forbes.com/sites/amymorin/2019/10/15/the-difference-between-helpful-problem-solving-and-harmful-overthinking/?sh=2fb195fa6e5f

Morin, A. (2023a, February 13). *How to be more confident: 9 tips that work.* Verywell Mind. https://www.verywellmind.com/how-to-boost-your-self-confidence-4163098

Morin, A. (2023b, February 14). *How to stop overthinking.* Verywell Mind. https://www.verywellmind.com/how-to-know-when-youre-overthinking-5077069

Neff, K. (2015, September 30). The five myths of self-compassion. *Greater Good Magazine.* https://greatergood.berkeley.edu/article/item/the_five_myths_of_self_compassion

Neff, K. (2020, July 9). *Definition of self-compassion.* Self-Compassion.org. https://self-compassion.org/the-three-elements-of-self-compassion-2/

Neff, K. (n.d.) Self-Compassion.org. https://self-compassion.org/

Never alone. (2022, March 21). *Overthinking quotes.* Never Alone. https://weareneveralone.co/blog/overthinking-quotes/

Newsonen, S. (2018, September 30). Why dogs make you happy. *Psychology Today*. https://www.psychologytoday.com/us/blog/the-path-passionate-happiness/201809/why-dogs-make-you-happy

Newman, K. (2021, March 31). *Unwinding your anxiety habit loop*. Mindful. https://www.mindful.org/unwinding-your-anxiety-habit-loop/

Nortje, A. (2020, May 14). *Mindful thinking: 4+ ways to stop ruminating & overthinking*. Positive Psychology. https://positivepsychology.com/mindful-thinking/

Oscar, D. (2022, January 5). *Why mindfulness is important*. Psychreg. https://www.psychreg.org/why-mindfulness-important/

Overthinking disorder: Is it a mental illness? (2022, December 9). Cleveland Clinic. https://health.clevelandclinic.org/is-overthinking-a-mental-illness/

Picoult, J. (2005). *My sister's keeper*. Washington Square Press. https://jodipicoult.com/my-sisters-keeper.html

Pinkler, S. (2020, December 30). Do dogs really make us happier? *The Wall Street Journal*. https://www.wsj.com/articles/do-dogs-really-make-us-happier-11609348272

Pittampalli, A. (2019, November 7). Why groups struggle to solve problems together. *Harvard Business Review*. https://hbr.org/2019/11/why-groups-struggle-to-solve-problems-together

Problem-solving: An essential soft skill to develop. (2022, October 13). Career Builder. https://www.careerbuilder.com/advice/blog/what-are-problemsolving-skills-and-why-are-they-important

PsychAlive. (2015, July 7). *Are you overthinking everything?* PsychAlive. https://www.psychalive.org/are-you-overthinking-everything/

Psychology Today Staff. (2022, January 4). Perfectionism. *Psychology Today*. https://www.psychologytoday.com/us/basics/perfectionism

Purche, W.R. (205). *Lessons to live by: The canine commandments*. Varzara House. https://www.amazon.com/Lessons-Live-Commandments-W-Pursche/dp/097537933X/ref=tmm_hrd_swatch_0?_encoding=UTF8&qid=1682028885&sr=8-2&tag=aurum0a-20

Roy, S. (2023, February 10). *How to stop overthinking (Get rid of overthinking the past)*. The Happiness Blog. https://happyproject.in/stop-overthinking/

Santilli, M. (2023, March 10). How to stop overthinking: Causes and ways to cope. *Forbes Health*. https://www.forbes.com/health/mind/what-causes-overthinking-and-6-ways-to-stop/

Schulz, C. (1962). *Happiness is a warm puppy*. Determined Productions, Inc. https://www.goodreads.com/book/show/1918249.Happiness_is_a_Warm_Puppy

Scott, E. (2022a, June 10). *How to overcome perfectionism*. Verywell Mind. https://www.verywellmind.com/overcoming-perfectionism-how-to-work-past-perfectionism-3144700

Scott, E. (2022b, December 30). *Effects of conflict and stress on relationships*. Verywell Mind. https://www.verywellmind.com/the-toll-of-conflict-in-relationships-3144952

Scott, E. (2023, February 27). *Perfectionism: 10 signs of perfectionist traits*. Verywell Mind. https://www.verywellmind.com/signs-you-may-be-a-perfectionist-3145233

Self-compassion vs. self-esteem. (2016, July 26). Center for Mindful Self-Compassion. https://centerformsc.org/learn-msc/self-compassion-vs-self-esteem/

Self-esteem and self-confidence. (2019, November 25). The University of Queensland Australia. https://my.uq.edu.au/information-and-services/student-support/health-and-wellbeing/self-help-resources/self-esteem-and-self-confidence

Smart, J. (2020, March 13). *How to improve your problem solving skills and build effective problem solving strategies*. Session Lab. https://www.sessionlab.com/blog/problem-solving-skills-and-strategies/

Sperber, S. (n.d.). *Overthinking: Definition, causes, & how to stop it*. Berkeley Well-Being Institute. https://www.berkeleywellbeing.com/overthinking.html

Stanborough, R. (2020, February 4). How to change negative thinking with cognitive restructuring. *Healthline.* https://www.healthline.com/health/cognitive-restructuring

Star, K. (2020, September 20). *How perfectionism can impact panic and anxiety.* Verywell Mind. https://www.verywellmind.com/perfectionism-and-panic-disorder-2584391

Stierwalt, S. (2018, December 17). Mindfulness: The science behind the practice. *Scientific American.* https://www.scientificamerican.com/article/mindfulness-the-science-behind-the-practice/

Stosny, S. (2014, February 26). *Do's and don'ts of self-compassion.* Psychology Today. https://www.psychologytoday.com/us/blog/anger-in-the-age-entitlement/201402/do-s-and-don-ts-self-compassion

Sutton, J. (n.d.). *Simple (4-column) thought diary worksheet.* Positive Psychology. https://positive.b-cdn.net/wp-content/uploads/2021/01/Simple-4-column-Thought-Diary-Worksheet.pdf

Sutton, J. (2017, April 3). *What is CBT? Defining cognitive behavioral therapy.* Positive Psychology. https://positivepsychology.com/what-is-cbt-definition-meaning/

Sutton, J. (2020a, June 19). *Socratic questioning in psychology: Examples and techniques.* Positive Psychology. https://positivepsychology.com/socratic-questioning/

Sutton, J. (2020b, July 15). *Why is mindfulness important? 20+ reasons to practice it today.* Positive Psychology. https://positivepsychology.com/importance-of-mindfulness/

Universal emotions. (2022, November 5). Paul Ekman Group. https://www.paulekman.com/universal-emotions/

Vale, R. (2013, March 15). The value of asking questions. *Molecular biology of the cell, 24*(6). https://www.molbiolcell.org/doi/10.1091/mbc.e12-09-0660

Vanbuskirk, S. (2023, February 21). *Why it's important to have high self-esteem.* Verywell Mind. https://www.verywellmind.com/why-it-s-important-to-have-high-self-esteem-5094127

Victorscorner. (2016, April 14). *16 powerful benefits of asking questions you should know*. Victors Corner. https://victorscorner.com/2016/04/14/benefits-of-asking-questions/

Ward, M. (2017, February 21). *14 methods to dramatically increase your self-confidence*. Cornerstone University. https://www.cornerstone.edu/blog-post/14-methods-to-dramatically-increase-your-self-confidence/

What is mindfulness? (n.d.). *Greater Good Magazine*. https://greatergood.berkeley.edu/topic/mindfulness/definition

Willard, C. (2021, December 15). *6 ways to enjoy mindful walking*. Mindful. https://www.mindful.org/6-ways-to-get-the-benefits-of-mindful-walking/

Williams, P., & Nussbaum, H. (2016, February 19). Chapter 21—Toward a neuroscience of wisdom. In *Neuroimaging personality, social cognition, and character* (pp. 383–395, J.R. Absher & J. Cloutier (Eds.)). Academic Press. https://www.sciencedirect.com/topics/psychology/emotional-stability

Zimmerman, M. A. (2013). Resiliency theory. *Health Education & Behavior*, *40*(4), 381–383. https://doi.org/10.1177/1090198113493782

Zolik, M-B. (2020, August 30). *Mindfulness for overthinking*. EMDR Healing. https://emdrhealing.com/mindfulness-for-overthinking/

HELPFUL RESOURCES

Centers for Disease Control and Prevention resources for people seeking help: https://www.cdc.gov/mentalhealth/tools-resources/individuals/index.htm

Cleveland Clinic, healthessentials@ccf.org, 9500 Euclid Ave., Cleveland, OH 44195, 1-800-223-2273

Emergency police, medical, fire: 911

Multidimensional Perfectionism Scale and Scoring https://hewittlab.sites.olt.ubc.ca/files/2014/11/MPS-RESEARCH-ONLY.pdf

National Alliance on Mental Illness (NAMI) Helpline 1-800-950-NAMI (6264) or https://nami.org

National Institute of Mental Health (NIMH) 1-866-615-6464, nimhinfo@nih.gov, or https://www.nimh.nih.gov/health/find-help

Substance Abuse and Mental Health Services Administration (SAMHSA) National Helpline 1-800-662-HELP (4357) or https://samhsa.gov

Suicide & Crisis Lifeline: 988 or https://988lifeline.org/